Biomechanics of Human Motion

Basics and Beyond
for the Health Professions

Biomechanics
of Human Motion

Basics and Beyond
for the Health Professions

BARNEY F. LEVEAU, PT, PhD
PROFESSOR, DEPARTMENT OF PHYSICAL THERAPY
COLLEGE OF HEALTH SCIENCES
ALABAMA STATE UNIVERSITY
MONTGOMERY, AL

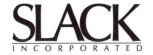

SLACK
INCORPORATED

The Instructor's Manual is also available from SLACK Incorporated. Don't miss this important companion to *Biomechanics of Human Motion: Basics and Beyond for the Health Professions*. To obtain the Instructor's Manual, please visit http://www.efacultylounge.com.

This book was published in a previous form by WB Saunders Company as *Biomechanics of Human Motion, Third Edition.*

Dr. Barney F. LeVeau has not disclosed any relevant financial relationships

The procedures and practices described in this book should be implemented in a manner consistent with the professional standards set for the circumstances that apply in each specific situation. Every effort has been made to confirm the accuracy of the information presented and to correctly relate generally accepted practices. The authors, editor, and publisher cannot accept responsibility for errors or exclusions or for the outcome of the material presented herein. There is no expressed or implied warranty of this book or information imparted by it. Care has been taken to ensure that drug selection and dosages are in accordance with currently accepted/recommended practice. Due to continuing research, changes in government policy and regulations, and various effects of drug reactions and interactions, it is recommended that the reader carefully review all materials and literature provided for each drug, especially those that are new or not frequently used. Any review or mention of specific companies or products is not intended as an endorsement by the author or publisher.

SLACK Incorporated uses a review process to evaluate submitted material. Prior to publication, educators or clinicians provide important feedback on the content that we publish. We welcome feedback on this work.

Published by: SLACK Incorporated
6900 Grove Road
Thorofare, NJ 08086 USA
Telephone: 856-848-1000
Fax: 856-853-5991
www.slackbooks.com

Contact SLACK Incorporated for more information about other b⋯⋯or about the availability of our books from distributors outside the United States.

Library of Congress Cataloging-in-Publication Data

LeVeau, Barney F. (Barney Francis), 1939-
  Biomechanics of human motion : basics and beyond for the health professions / Barney F. LeVeau.
       p. ; cm.
  Includes bibliographical references and index.
  ISBN 978-1-55642-905-7 (alk. paper)
  1. Human mechanics. 2. Biomechanics. I. Title.
  [DNLM: 1. Movement. 2. Biomechanics. WE 103 L657b 2010]
  QP303.L48 2010
  612.7'6--dc22
                              2010012720

Last digit is print number: 10 9 8 7 6 5 4 3 2 1

7450617

DEDICATION

To my parents who, although they were share croppers and had limited formal education, worked extra jobs to provide opportunities and encouragement for all of their children to obtain postgraduate degrees.

Contents

ACKNOWLEDGMENTS

I would like to thank the Mechanical Kinesiology classes at Alabama State University who gave criticism and support for the development of this edition. I would like to thank my wife for her patience as I took time away from vacations and weekends with her.

I would also like to thank Brien Cummings, Dani Karaszkiewicz, Debra Toulson, Michael Bress, and Donna Trapani for their assistance in preparation of this book.

ABOUT THE AUTHOR

Dr. LeVeau earned his BS degree in Education with emphasis in mathematics, physics, and physical education at the University of Colorado in Boulder, CO; his Certificate in Physical Therapy from the Mayo Clinic in Rochester, MN; his MS in Physical Education from the University of Colorado; and his PhD in Biomechanics from Pennsylvania State University in University Park, PA.

He has taught mathematics and science at Horace Mann Jr. High School in Colorado Springs, CO, and served as faculty in physical education and physical therapy departments at West Chester State College in West Chester, PA; University of North Carolina at Chapel Hill, NC; University of Texas Southwestern Medical Center at Dallas, TX; Georgia State University in Atlanta, GA; and Alabama State University in Montgomery, AL.

He has published several research articles, book chapters, and 2 textbook editions related to biomechanics content. His texts have been translated in Spanish, French, and Italian. He has lectured nationally and internationally on topics covering biomechanics.

INTRODUCTION

The focus of this book is on force. Force is always with you. Force is involved with large objects, such as the interaction among the sun, moon, and earth, or in very small objects, such as interactions among cells. Many disciplines are involved in the study of force and its effects on objects. This book will provide a basic background for many of these disciplines, including exercise science, physical therapy, occupational therapy, sports medicine, prosthetics and orthotics, orthopedics, rehabilitation medicine, dentistry, veterinary medicine, and ergonomics. Some areas of study relevant to biomechanics include anatomy, growth process, external loads, trauma, ergonomics, clinical evaluation, clinical treatment, protective equipment, prosthetics, orthotics, and body movement.

The purpose of this book is to present the basic principles of biomechanics and to provide techniques and examples for approaching biomechanical situations. Based upon the concept of force, the book illustrates how force is applied to the human body and how the body applies force to various objects. The emphasis is on the pertinent factors that guide the reader to an understanding of biomechanics at a beginning level. The recent articles listed at the end of each chapter should provide the reader with information beyond the basics.

When studying mechanics, you will become involved with mathematical formulas. Don't be afraid of formulas. They are just a shorthand method for writing definitions and showing relationships among variables. You should remember the units for each variable. You can then use unit analysis to show relationships.

Various disciplines do not use the same system of units. Although the International System of Units (SI) has become widely accepted, its use by practitioners in the United States is still not widespread. Practitioners and clinicians are more likely to use the English measurement system, while researchers and scientists rely on the SI system. Because this is a basic text, the English system will be presented. However, the conversion table in the appendix will allow the reader to convert units from English to SI and SI to English with little difficulty. By using the conversion table and unit analysis, for example, you may convert miles per hour (mph) to meters per second (m/sec) or (msec-1).

55 mph x 1 hr/60 min x 1 min/60 sec x 5280 ft/1 mi x 0.3048 m/1 ft = 24.587 m/sec

The units of miles, hours, minutes, and feet all cancel out, leaving the units of m/sec.

The problems in the text should not be considered exact. Several assumptions occur when we attempt to determine force acting on the body or the body acting on an object. In this text:

1. Only 2-dimensional figures are used.

2. Calculations of muscle force often refer to a muscle group and not necessarily the force of a single muscle.

3. The mass and weight of body segments are estimates based upon reported research. (See Appendix.)

4. The lengths of lever arms are estimates based upon reported research. (See Appendix.)

5. The minimal amount of friction in the joints is disregarded.

6. Effects of ligaments, synergists, antagonists, co-contractions, and other soft tissues are disregarded in the calculations.

An Instructor's Manual has been developed that provides questions and problems for worksheets, quizzes, and examinations.

chapter 1

Force

Objectives

1. Present and discuss examples of biomechanics in the clinic and everyday life.
2. Define basic terms.
3. Draw and label the 4 characteristics of a force.
4. Describe and give examples of 8 types of force.
5. Describe an exercise for each type of force.
6. Differentiate isometric, concentric, and eccentric contractions.
7. Discuss the concept of pressure.
8. Relate mass and moment of inertia.
9. Relate the concepts of energy, work, and power.
10. Explain Newton's 3 laws.

Definition, Description, and Scope

Biomechanics is the study of forces and their effect on living organisms. It is basic to the understanding of human movement; mechanics of injury; and the principles of prevention, evaluation, and treatment of musculoskeletal problems. Concepts of biomechanics are not limited to the study of the range of motion of joints, posture, and analysis of locomotion or gait. Everything we do involves biomechanics in some form or degree. The principles of biomechanics are at work in the "couch potato" as well as the elite athlete. Biomechanical principles apply to disabled as well as able-bodied individuals. They are employed throughout the lifespan from the womb until death. Because biomechanics is the study of the effect of forces on the human body, whenever a force is present, biomechanical principles are involved.

Biomechanics applies principles and concepts that are very important to the disciplines including exercise science, physical therapy, occupational therapy, sports medicine, prosthetics and orthotics, orthopedics, rehabilitation medicine, podiatry, dentistry, and veterinary medicine. These are health professionals who use biomechanical concepts to evaluate and treat patients and to improve motor performance. In addition, professionals such as bioengineers, ergonomists, and human factors specialists use biomechanical concepts to understand how individuals physically interact with their environments (eg, the workplace, vehicles, and tools) and to explore the efficiency and safety with which this interaction takes place.

LeVeau BF.
Biomechanics of Human Motion: Basics and Beyond for the Health Professions (pp 1-34).
© 2011 SLACK Incorporated

Biomechanics is based on the content areas of anatomy, physiology, motor learning, mathematics, physics, and clinical sciences. This basic knowledge level allows the individual to understand how forces and anatomy interrelate. A general course in biomechanics can serve as a foundation for both clinical and sports-related biomechanics. Individuals with more advanced knowledge will be able to analyze and evaluate how forces specifically act on the body and how the body exerts forces on other objects. They will also be able to research and establish programs to enhance rehabilitation and prevent injuries. The advanced biomechanist will be able to design an environment that allows disabled individuals to live an efficient and safer lifestyle and possibly to participate in recreational and competitive sporting activities.

Additional content areas in biomechanics include specific rehabilitation techniques, wheelchair design, anthropology, specific tissue repair, surgical techniques, and architecture. Because force, the basis of biomechanics, is everywhere, the scope of biomechanics is only limited by one's imagination and the needs of specific populations.

The biomechanist must know how the body responds in normal situations in order to set goals for the injured or disabled individual. The biomechanist must understand the specific activities of the individual in order to help prevent injuries from occurring. Normal patterns of movement and their variations for healthy individuals must be understood in order for the movement pattern of an injured or disabled individual to be directed toward a more normal pattern. If movement cannot return to normal, the movement pattern must be directed toward the most efficient and safe pattern for that individual. To analyze these movement patterns, the biomechanist uses instrumentation and techniques, such as video analysis, electromyography (EMG), electrogoniometry (elgon), accelerometry, and force plate and force transducer analysis.

Force

Force is an important concept to grasp in studying biomechanics. Forces can be separated, combined, and manipulated. An understanding of how force acts on objects and what can result when forces are applied to various materials is central to the study of biomechanics.

Force can be defined simply as a push or pull. Force can be considered as the entity that tends to produce motion, to halt motion, or to change the direction of motion. When motion occurs, force is the factor that causes a mass to accelerate. This relationship is depicted in the equation $F = ma$. F stands for force; m stands for mass of the object; and a represents the acceleration (+ or -) of the object. This formula may be rearranged to be $a = \frac{F}{m}$. This formula represents Newton's Second Law of Motion or the law of acceleration. Acceleration of an object is directly proportional to the force applied and inversely proportional to its mass.

Force is a vector quantity (has magnitude and direction) and not scalar (has only magnitude). To define force, however, it must be described by 4 characteristics: point of application, line of application, direction of pull or push, and magnitude (Figure 1-1). Force must have a point of application. Examples of points of application are contact between bones at joints, attachments of muscles to bones, the center of mass of a limb, and the point of contact of a dumbbell (Figure 1-2). Force acts anywhere along a line of application, but this line can be redirected by a fixed pulley. For example, the peroneus longus tendon traversing behind the lateral malleolus provides an example inside the body of a fixed pulley changing the line of application of the force produced by a muscle (Figure 1-3). The third characteristic of force is its direction of pull or push. In Figure 1-1, an arrowhead placed at the end of the line of application shows the direction of the force. The force of gravity, for example, provides a downward direction on the human body. Magnitude, which is the quantity of force, is the fourth characteristic of a force. Every force

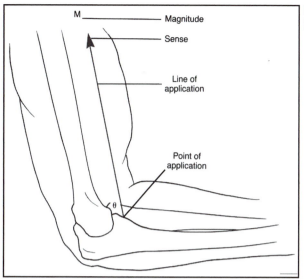

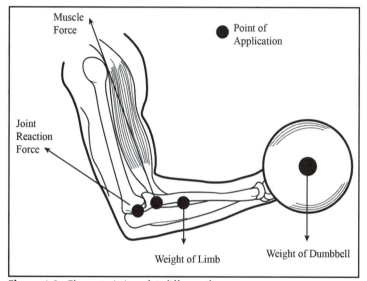

Figure 1-1. A force vector and the 4 characteristics of force.

Figure 1-2. Characteristics of 4 different forces.

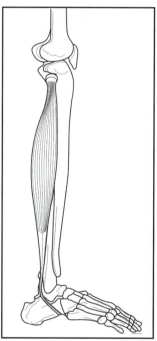

Figure 1-3. The lateral malleolus as a pulley.

has these 4 characteristics, and all 4 characteristics must be considered when studying a force or forces. The unit of force is the Newton or pound.

Types of Force

Several types of forces exist. Some scientists classify forces into only 2 categories: contact forces and action-at-a-distance (non-contact) forces. Others consider the natural forces as gravitational, electromagnetic, strong nuclear, and weak nuclear. In this text, we will address the forces that are common to the health and exercise professional. These forces include gravitational, contact, frictional, muscular, inertial, elastic, buoyant, and electromagnetic.

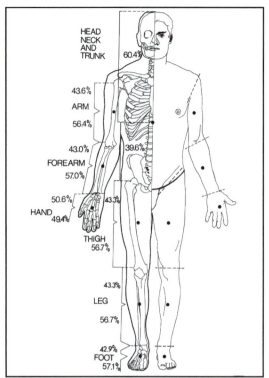

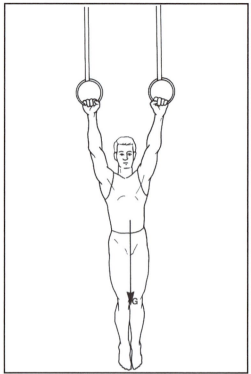

Figure 1-4. Link boundaries (at the joint centers) and percentage distance of centers of gravity from link boundaries. (Data from Dempster WT. *Space Requirements of the Seated Operator: Geometrical, Kinematic, and Mechanical Aspects of the Body, With Special Reference to the Limbs.* Dayton, OH: WADC Technical Report 55-159; 1955.)

Figure 1-5. Gravity acting on a gymnast's body.

GRAVITATIONAL

The force of gravity, usually considered the most common force, is the mutual attraction between 2 objects. The magnitude of the force of gravity is directly proportional to the mass of each object and inversely proportional to the distance between the objects.

$$F_g = \frac{Gm_1m_2}{r^2}$$

Because the mass of the earth is extremely large, the earth dominates over the negligible attraction between other objects. The magnitude of the earth's gravity on an object is called its weight (W). The following equations illustrate the relationship between weight and mass and can be shown as $F = ma$, or $W = mg$, where m is the mass of the object and g is the acceleration of the object caused by the earth's gravitational force (32.2 ft/sec^2 or 9.81 m/sec^2).

Although an object is usually made up of several small components, the point of application is considered to be the center of mass of the object. The weight of the arm or leg, for example, is considered to be concentrated at the center of mass of the body part (Figure 1-4). The line of application of the gravitational force is a straight line between the center of mass of the 2 objects. For the earth, this line is vertical. Of the 2 objects attracting each other, the one that is most easily moved travels toward the less moveable object. Hence, on earth, all objects are directed toward the center of the earth, which we call "down" (Figure 1-5).

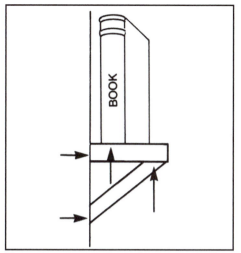

Figure 1-6. Contact force: book on a shelf.

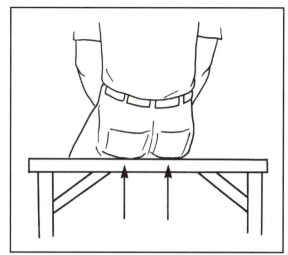

Figure 1-7. Contact force: person sitting on a bench.

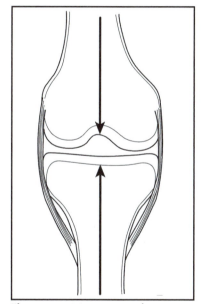

Figure 1-8. Joint reaction force.

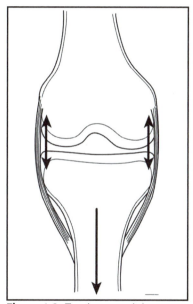

Figure 1-9. Tension on a joint.

CONTACT

Whenever 2 objects are in contact, a force exists between them (Figures 1-6 and 1-7). A contact force is the result of an outside or external force, called a load. Contact forces are related to Newton's Third Law or law of reaction. That is, for every force that is applied, there is a force acting with equal magnitude in the opposite direction.

An important but often overlooked contact force is the joint reaction force (Figure 1-8). Forces acting on bones can set up contact forces in the joints that can cause compression of the articular cartilage and underlying ends of the involved bones. In some situations, distraction (pulling apart) occurs at the joint (Figure 1-9). Hence, ligaments and other soft tissues are placed under tension while the compression on the cartilage and bone is reduced. Contact forces are very common and exist in all postures and movements.

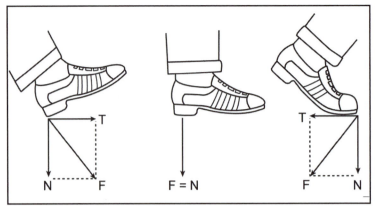

Figure 1-10. Friction during locomotion: F represents contact force, N represents normal force, T represents tangential or frictional force.

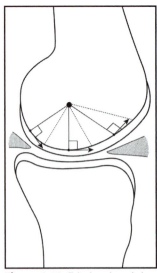

Figure 1-11. Friction in a joint.

FRICTIONAL

If movement occurs between 2 solid objects in contact, friction develops. The magnitude of frictional force (F_s) depends upon the composition of the adjacent surfaces. The 2 surfaces establish the coefficient of friction (μ), which is the ratio between the force of friction and the normal force (N). The normal force is the force component that is perpendicular to the supporting surface. A greater force of contact during the movement produces a greater frictional force. The coefficient of friction times the normal force between the 2 surfaces equals the force (F_s) created by friction:

$$F_s = \mu N$$

A high contact force with movement can produce tissue damage. Examples of such damage are degenerative joint disease of the hip, patellofemoral joint syndrome, and lacerations of the hands in gymnastics. Friction is involved in locomotion (Figure 1-10), in prosthetic devices, in joint motion (Figure 1-11), and in various exercise devices (Figures 1-12 and 1-13).

Another example of friction is the concept of "fluid friction" or viscosity. Viscosity is the internal resistance to the flow of a fluid. As a fluid flows through a tube or pipe, friction between the wall of the tube and the fluid retards the flow of the fluid. Layers of fluid molecules move past each other (laminar flow) creating friction between these layers. This viscosity, or fluid friction, creates a resisting force that requires a force to be exerted to cause one layer of fluid to slide past the other (Figure 1-14). As an object moves through a fluid, friction is produced between the object and the fluid. This friction encountered by the object moving through the fluid depends on the viscosity of the fluid, the size and shape of the object, and the velocity of the object. An object with weight, W, sinking in a fluid is retarded in its movement by buoyancy, B, and friction, F (Figure 1-15).

MUSCULAR

Muscle force is an important force for the maintenance of body posture and movement (Figure 1-16). In general, muscles function as motors, providing the force that moves our appendicular skeleton and helps to assume and maintain certain postures, and to hold us up (Figure 1-17).

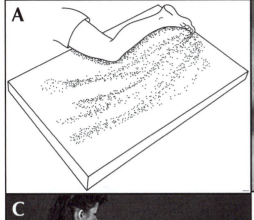

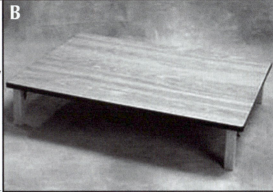

Figure 1-12. (B) Powderboard table and (C) Powderboard. Reprinted with permission from Patterson Medical/Sammons Preston, Bolingbrook, IL.

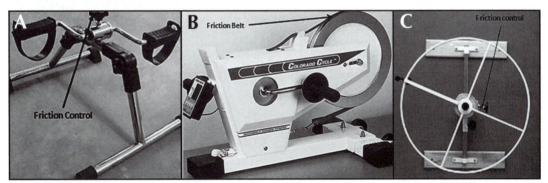

Figure 1-13. Friction in exercise devices. Reprinted with permission from Patterson Medical/Sammons Preston, Bolingbrook, IL.

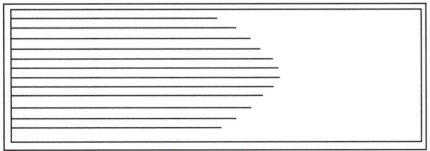

Figure 1-14. Friction in fluid flow.

Figure 1-15. Object sinking in a fluid: W represents the object's weight; B represents buoyancy force; and F represents the force of friction between object and water.

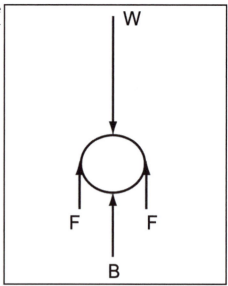

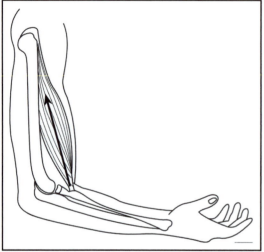

Figure 1-16. Muscle force.

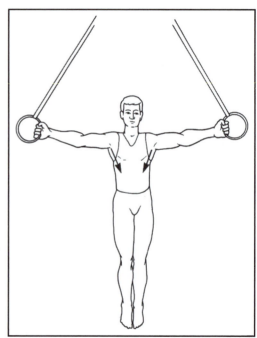

Figure 1-17. The use of muscle force to overcome gravity and move the body.

Muscles have the properties of excitability, conductivity, contractility, extensibility, and elasticity and are capable of producing force under the control of the nervous system. The excitability of a muscle gives it the ability to respond to a stimulus. Conductivity gives it the ability to propagate an electrical current. Contractility is the ability of the muscle to shorten and generate force when an adequate stimulus is received. The muscle can be stretched (extensibility) and then returned to its original resting length (elasticity) when the stretching force is removed. The magnitude of force that a muscle can produce depends upon its contractile ability, its structure, and its biomechanical/biochemical characteristics.

Figure 1-18. Motor unit with nerve and associated muscle fibers.

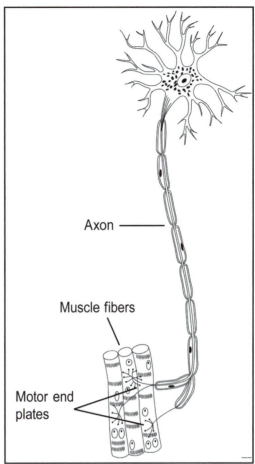

Axon

Muscle fibers

Motor end plates

The contractile ability and structure of the muscle influence the magnitude of force that a muscle can produce. The contractile ability of the muscle depends upon the rate of motor unit firing, the number of motor units firing, and the size of the motor units. A motor unit consists of the nerve and all of the muscle fibers that connect to it (Figure 1-18). The muscle's contractile ability and the magnitude of force it can develop also depends upon its physiological cross-sectional area, the length of the muscle, its type of contraction, and its speed of contraction (Table 1-1).

A direct relationship exists between the length of a muscle and the magnitude of force it can produce (Figures 1-19 and 1-20). The position of the actin and myosin filaments of the muscle fibers helps to determine the amount of force generated. Muscle develops maximal force when the actin and myosin filaments (the contractile proteins of muscle) are arranged to form the maximum number of connections, or cross-bridges. If the muscle is made longer or shorter than this optimal length, fewer cross-bridges are formed, and less force develops. When the muscle is sufficiently stretched, actin and myosin filaments are positioned sufficiently apart so that all connections or cross-bridges cannot form. As the muscle is shortened, the actin and myosin filaments overlap, and additional cross-bridges are formed. At the position (optimal length) where the greatest overlapping region for filaments is obtained, the greatest magnitude of force occurs. As the muscle is placed in a shorter position, the actin and myosin filaments tend to overlap themselves, which reduces the number of cross-bridges that can be formed.

TABLE 1-1

Contractile Ability of Muscle

• Rate of motor unit firing • Number of motor units firing • Size of motor units • Cross-section area	• Muscle length • Type of contraction • Speed of contraction

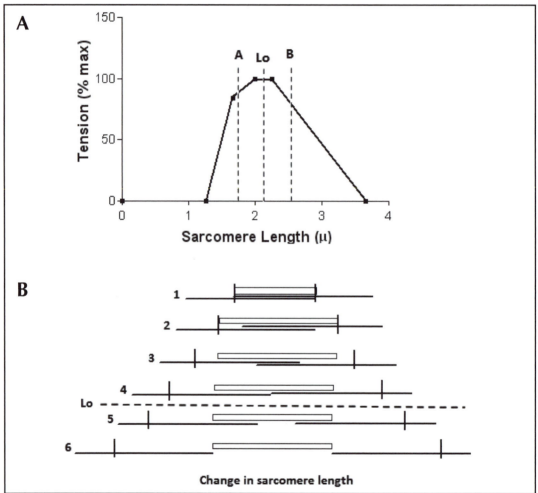

Figure 1-19. Length-tension relationship for sarcomere shortening adapted from data from Gordon AM, Huxley AF, Julian FJ. The variation in isometric tension with sarcomere length in vertebrate muscle fibres. *J Physiol.* 1966;184:170-92; Cutts A. The range of sarcomere lengths in the muscles of the human lower limb. *J Anat.* 1988;160:79-88; and Reeves ND, Narici MV, Maganaris CN. In vivo human muscle structure and function: adaptations to resistance training in old age. *Experimental Physiology.* 2004;89:675-689. (A) Lo is considered to be the optimal sarcomere length. The space between A and B is the estimated normal operating range of the sarcomere. (B) Lo is considered to be the optimal sarcomere length. In a representation of relationship between thick and thin filaments, 4 and 5 are within the estimated normal operating range of the sarcomere; 1 is when the Z lines compress the thick filaments resisting shortening; and 6 when the sarcomere is lengthened so that no overlap of the filaments exist.

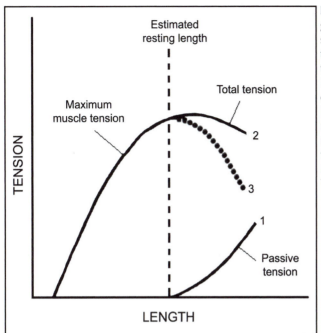

Figure 1-20. Isometric length-tension diagram for striated muscle. If passive tension curve (line 1) is subtracted from total tension curve (line 2), maximum muscle tension is developed at the normal resting length of muscle (line 3). The resting length of muscle is about 20% longer than the length of an excised, completely relaxed muscle. The horizontal axis represents muscle length; the vertical axis represents force. (Adapted from Astrand PO, Rodahl K. *Textbook of Work Physiology.* New York, NY: McGraw-Hill; 1970.)

The velocity of muscle shortening has a predictable effect upon the force that a muscle can produce (Figure 1-21). Because cross-bridges require a minimum of time to attach and develop force, their function is dependent upon the rate of shortening. As the filaments slide past each other at a faster rate, fewer cross-bridges can be formed at a specific instant. Thus, as a muscle shortens faster, the magnitude of force produced is decreased. Even during a contraction with no change in muscle length, a brief time is needed for a muscle to develop its full force. This phenomenon is illustrated by the force-time curve shown in Figure 1-22.

Force is produced by a muscle whenever cross-bridges are formed. If the muscle force that is developed is equal to the resistance offered at the attachments of the muscle, and no change in length of the total muscle occurs, the type of muscle contraction is isometric. If the muscle force results in a change in length of the total muscle, the contraction is considered to be isotonic and is either concentric or eccentric. A concentric contraction occurs if the muscle force exceeds the resistance offered at the muscle attachments and the distance between the attachments decreases. An eccentric contraction occurs when the resisting force at the muscle attachments exceeds the muscle force produced by the muscle and the muscle lengthens. An eccentric contraction can control a greater magnitude of external force than an isometric contraction (Figure 1-23). In turn, an isometric contraction can hold a greater magnitude of external force than a concentric contraction (see Figure 1-23).

The number of motor units that are active in the different types of contractions shows the reverse order (Figure 1-24). If the same resistance is applied, the concentric contraction requires a greater number of active motor units than an isometric contraction. An isometric contraction uses more active motor units than an eccentric contraction.

Inertial

Whether an object is stationary or moving, it has the property of inertia. As stated in Newton's First Law or law of inertia, an object at rest tends to remain at rest, and an object in motion tends

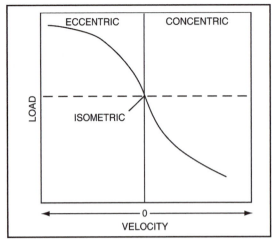

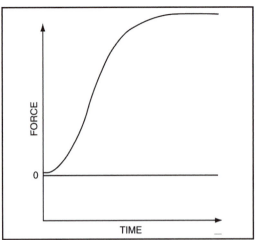

Figure 1-21. Force-velocity curve for elbow flexor muscles. (Adapted from Komi PV. Measurement of the force-velocity relationship in human muscle under concentric and eccentric contractions. In Cerquiglini S, Venerando S, Wartenweiler J, eds. *Biomechanics III*. Baltimore, MD: University Park Press; 1973:227.)

Figure 1-22. Force-time curve for human muscle. (Adapted from Stotthart JP. Relationship between selected biomechanical parameters of static and dynamic performance. In Cerquiglini S, Venerando S, Wartenweiler J, eds. *Biomechanics III*. Baltimore, MD: University Park Press; 1973:212.)

Figure 1-23. Curves of maximum eccentric, isometric, and concentric forces of forearm flexors. (Reprinted with permission from the American Physiological Society. Figure 2 from M. Singh and P. V. Karpovich. Isotonic and isometric forces of forearm flexors and extensors. *J Appl Physiol.* 21(4):1435-1437, 1966.)

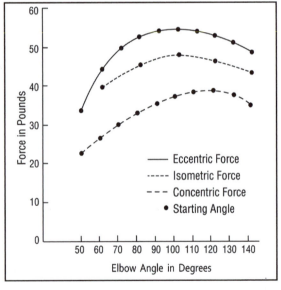

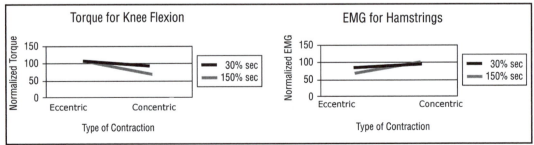

Figure 1-24. Maximum knee flexion resultant joint moment at 30 degrees and 150 degrees per second compared to normalized electromyographic activity of the hamstring muscles. (Based on data from Kellis E, Baltzopoulis V. Muscle activation differences between eccentric and concentric isokinetic exercise. *Med Sci Sports Exerc.* 1998;30(11):1616-1623.)

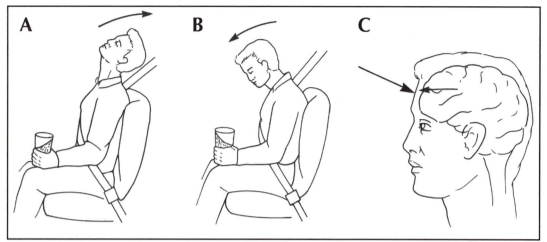

Figure 1-25. Effects of inertia. (A) If an automobile starts rapidly or is hit from behind, the head tends to remain at rest as the body is moved forward. (B) If an automobile stops rapidly, the head tends to continue moving as the body stops (note the fluid level in the cup). (C) The inertia of the brain can cause brain and vessel damage if the head is hit or stopped suddenly.

to remain in motion at a constant velocity unless acted upon by an external force. This law indicates that inertia is a force that resists an object's change in movement status. A force external to the object must be applied to a stationary object to make it move or to a moving object to make it stop or change direction. This change in the status of motion changes the velocity of the object. The change in velocity, whether positive or negative, is called acceleration or deceleration, respectively.

The magnitude needed by an external force of an object to start, stop, or change its direction is determined by the equation $F = ma$. The line of application of the inertial force for a moving object is along its straight path of motion. The force is directed along the same line as the moving object. The point of application is considered to be at the object's center of mass. Some examples of inertia include the motion of a driver's head when the automobile stops, starts, or is hit from the rear (Figure 1-25); starting, stopping, or changing direction of a large, heavily loaded truck; and the starting, stopping, or changing direction of an exercise weight. Inertia is involved with all exercise devices because it resists change in motion. The Impulse Inertial Exercise Trainer (Impulse Training Systems, Newnan, GA) uses inertia as its primary resistance for exercise (Figure 1-26).

Elastic

Some materials have the capacity to return to their original size and shape once they have been deformed. In elastic materials, the amount of deformation is directly proportional to the force used to deform the material (Hooke's Law). This type of force is called *elastic force*. The magnitude of the force depends upon the type of material and the amount of deformation ($F = -kl$), with k representing a constant value for the specific type of material and l representing the amount of deformation that has occurred. The line of application is along the line of the deforming force, but acts in the opposite direction. The point of application is the point of contact between the elastic material and the external force. Strengthening devices have been developed that use elastic force as the resisting force, such as elastic bands (Figure 1-27A), sponge balls (Figure 1-27B), and bending rods (Figure 1-27C). Splints (Figure 1-28) and orthoses may have an elastic component involved in their construction.

Figure 1-26. The Impulse Inertial Exercise Trainer is based upon the use of inertial force for resistance. (Courtesy of Impulse Training Systems, Newnan, GA).

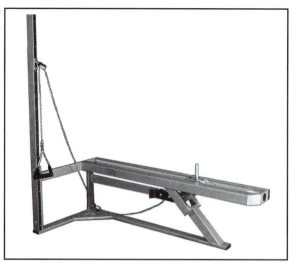

Figure 1-27. Elastic force as a resisting force. (A) Elastic band. (B) Thera-Band Hand Exerciser. (C) Digi-Extend Finger Exerciser. (D) Bowflex Ultimate. Reprinted with permission from Patterson Medical/Sammons Preston, Bolingbrook, IL.

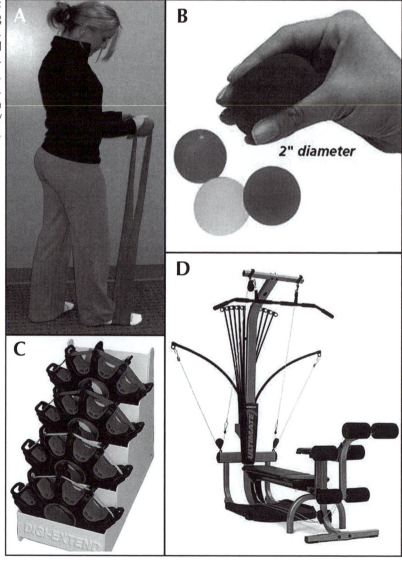

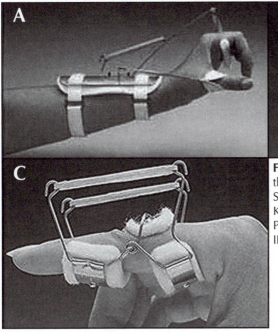

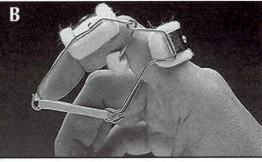

Figure 1-28. Splints use elastic force as part of their construction. (A) Bunnell Thomas Suspension Splint. (B) Reverse Finger Knuckle Bender. (C) Finger Knuckle Bender. Reprinted with permission from Patterson Medical/Sammons Preston, Bolingbrook, IL.

BUOYANT

An upward, buoyant force acts upon an object when that object is immersed in a fluid, with the magnitude of the force equal to the weight of the fluid displaced by the object (Figure 1-29). The line of application of the buoyant force is vertical, and the effective point of application is at the object's center of mass. Because of the buoyant force of water, pool therapy is often used to reduce the force of gravity on the lower limbs. While an individual is standing in the pool, the force (F) on the individual's feet is equal to the body weight (W) minus the weight of the water displaced (B), or $F = W - B$. The buoyant force reduces the load on lower limbs as the individual is standing in a pool (Figures 1-30 and 1-31).

ELECTROMAGNETIC (EDDY CURRENTS)

A force field called a magnetic field exists in the space surrounding a magnet, a moving charge, and a wire carrying a current. Materials such as iron, nickel, cobalt, or their alloys have the internal domains of atoms that can be aligned to produce a magnetic field.

A magnetic field can also be produced around a wire carrying a current. The magnetic force is caused by electrons in motion. If the wire is coiled, a focused magnetic field is established similar to that of a bar magnet. This field is made stronger by placing an iron-like material through the center of the coil. This process creates an electromagnet. The magnitude of the magnetic force is proportional to the magnitude of the electrical current, to the number of turns or coils, and to the use of an iron core. Many devices in modern technology depend upon electromagnetism, including door bells, electric clocks, and telephones.

An electric current may be induced into a conductor as relative motion occurs between the conductor and the magnetic field. Usually, the conductor is a wire with either the wire moving in a magnetic field or the field moving and the conductor stationary. The magnitude of the electrical current produced depends upon the strength of the magnetic field and the velocity of the relative motion.

Figure 1-29. Buoyancy.

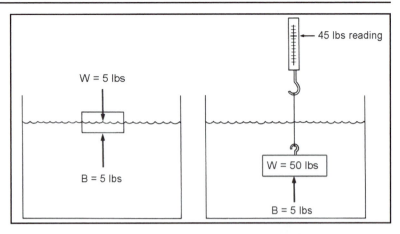

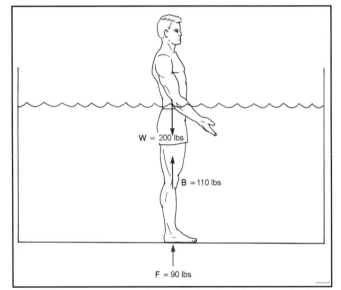

Figure 1-30. Buoyancy: reducing the load on the lower limb.

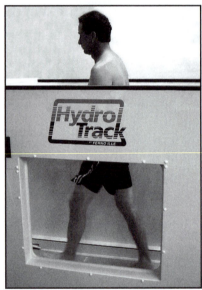

Figure 1-31. Buoyancy: walking on a treadmill in water. (© Ferno Aquatic Therapy, Wilmington, OH.)

Electromagnetic induction also occurs in a conducting material, such as a metal plate or disc, when it is moved through a magnetic field. In this situation, the conducting material is not connected to a circuit. When the plate or disc moves through the magnetic field, electric currents circulate within the material. These electric currents rotate in closed loops like whirlpools (Figure 1-32). These induced currents, called eddy currents, produce magnetic fields that oppose the motion of the conducting material.

Suppose a metal disc rotates in a magnetic field that is perpendicular to the plane of the disc and that covers only a small portion of the area of the disc. Eddy currents are established within the disc in the area of the magnetic field. The eddy currents oppose the motion of the disc and act as a breaking action on the disc (eddy current braking or damping). The greater the area of interaction (Figure 1-32B and 1-32C), the greater the braking action becomes. The braking effect is similar to friction without the contact and mechanical wearing. Mechanical work must be applied to the disc to keep it rotating at a constant velocity. This concept of magnetic braking is used in brakes for railroad trains, amusement park rides, and in exercise devices such as stationary bicycles, steppers, rowing machines, and elliptical devices.

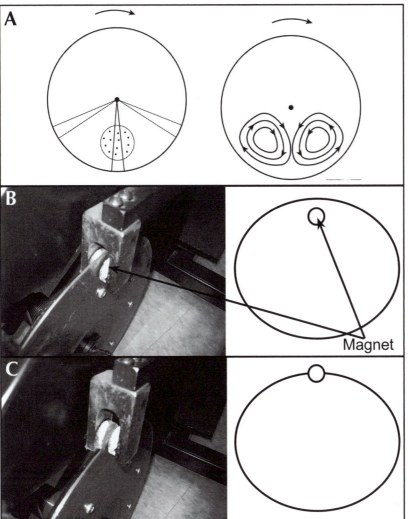

Figure 1-32. Electromagnetic force as resistance for exercise devices. (B) High resistance. (C) Less resistance.

Related Terms

TORQUE

Force acting at a distance from the pivot point of a lever produces torque or a moment of force (Figure 1-33). A moment of force (T) has the tendency to cause rotation about an axis. It is equal to the magnitude of force (F) multiplied by the perpendicular distance from the line of application of the force to the axis (d), or

$$T = F \times d$$

STRENGTH

The term strength is used 2 different ways in the discipline of biomechanics. The first concept of strength is related to the muscular type of force. Muscular strength is the ability of the muscle to produce or resist force. The second concept of strength is related to the elastic type of force. The strength of a material is the ability of the material or object to resist deformation.

Figure 1-33. Torque or moment of force.

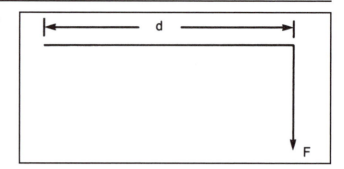

LOAD

An outside force or combination of forces applied externally to an object is called a load. An individual sitting on a bench applies a load to the bench, to the soft tissue of the buttocks area, and to the ischial tuberosities (Figure 1-34). A weight in the hand provides a load to many structures in the arm (Figure 1-35). A muscle pulling on its bony attachment puts a load on the bone. Lying in bed places loads on each calcaneus, on the sacrum, on each scapula, and on the occiput, as well as on soft tissues of the body.

PRESSURE

Pressure is the result of a contact force. As a load is applied to an object, the load is distributed over an area of the object. Pressure indicates how this force is distributed. Pressure is defined as the total force per area over which the force is applied. This can be shown by the following equation: Pressure (P) equals the Force (F) divided by the Area (A), or

$$P = \frac{F}{A}$$

This formula provides the average pressure of force per unit area (for example, pounds per square inch, Newtons per square meter, or Pascals). A force acting over a large area produces less pressure than the same force acting over a small area (Figure 1-36).

Example: If the pad of a brace exerts a 4 lb force over an area of 6 in by 8 in, the average pressure between the pad and the skin would be 4 divided by 48 in^2, or about 0.083 lb per in^2.

$$P = \frac{F}{A}$$

$$P = \frac{4 \text{ lb}}{(6 \text{ in x } 8 \text{ in})}$$

$$P = \frac{4 \text{ lb}}{48 \text{ in}^2}$$

$$P = 0.083 \text{ lb/in}^2$$

Pressure ulcers are a major problem confronting the severely disabled or debilitated patient. Pressure ulcers prolong the patient's morbidity and interfere with rehabilitation. Ulceration of the skin occurs, especially over a bony prominence when the patient is subjected to long periods of immobilization, and the pressure from the body weight exceeds the capillary pressure. These pressure ulcers, however, are preventable. Pressure can be reduced by either decreasing the force, increasing the area over which the force is acting, or both. A soft boot over the foot will spread the load of the foot over a larger area than the bony calcaneus and reduce the chance of pressure sores developing (Figure 1-37).

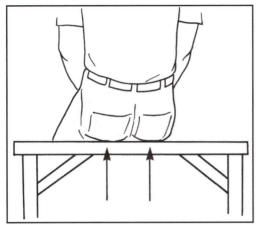

Figure 1-34. Load on the ischial tuberosities.

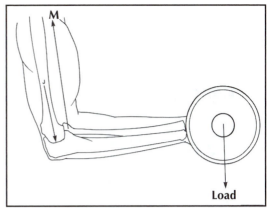

Figure 1-35. Load in the hand.

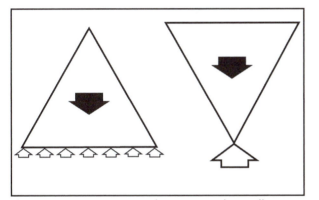

Figure 1-36. Pressure over a large area and a small area.

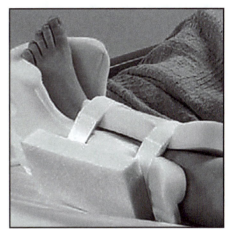

Figure 1-37. Reduction of pressure using a Heel Lift Traction Boot. Reprinted with permission from Patterson Medical/Sammons Preston, Bolingbrook, IL.

Fluids in an Open Container

Pressure is an important concept in the use of fluids. As the force of gravity acts on a fluid at rest, it will pull the fluid toward the center of the earth, producing a pressure within the fluid and between the fluid and its supporting container. The pressure on an object within the fluid depends upon the magnitude of the weight of the fluid above the object. As an object descends in a fluid, the pressure on the object will increase. The pressure of a fluid at a specific depth in a container depends upon the depth of the object at that point and density of the fluid, but is not affected by the shape of the container (Figure 1-38). Air pressure changes at different altitudes in airplanes or driving over mountain passes can be felt in the ears. Pressure in water changes during scuba diving and snorkeling. This change in pressure can cause pain and medical problems.

As a diver descends deeper under the surface of the water, the hydrostatic pressure increases (Figure 1-39). The pressure at any given depth in a fluid depends upon the density of the fluid. Hence, the pressure in water (hydraulic pressure) is much greater than in air (atmospheric pressure).

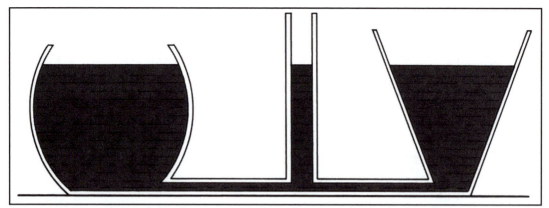

Figure 1-38. The pressure of a fluid in a container depends only on the depth of the fluid and not upon the shape of the container.

Figure 1-39. Pressure on the diver is the same at all points at depth y. As y increases, the pressure also increases.

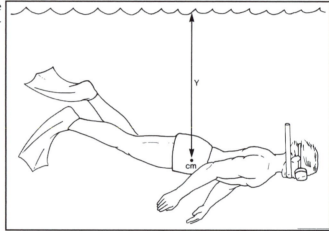

Fluids in a Closed Container

Because of the ability of a gas to completely fill an enclosed container, a gas will exert pressure on all sides of the container. According to Pascal's Law, this pressure is applied equally to all parts of the container. When more gas is added to the container, the density and pressure of the gas increase. Gases are highly compressible.

A compressed gas is assumed to be perfectly elastic and has the properties of Hooke's Law and resilience. These properties are used in automobile tires, balls, balloons, and other objects whose size and shapes are maintained by compressed air.

Similarly, when a force is applied to an enclosed liquid, the force is transmitted equally to every portion of the fluid and to every part of the container. Liquids can be considered to be incompressible. Pascal's Law is also applied to liquids. Hence, the pressure in a liquid will be transmitted equally throughout the container without a change in volume. This pressure will be transmitted instantaneously in an incompressible liquid. An example of such pressure in the human body is the fluid within the intervertebral disc (Figure 1-40). These concepts are the basis of hydraulics. Hydraulic lifts (Figure 1-41), hydraulic brakes, and hydraulic exercise devices are related to this principle. In contrast, a delay in the transmission of pressure occurs in a compressible fluid. The pressure changes at the speed of sound throughout the fluid. Gases are examples of compressible fluids, and pneumatics is the study of the properties of compressed air.

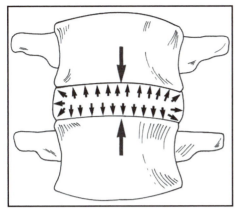

Figure 1-40. Pressure within an intervertebral disc resulting from load on a disc.

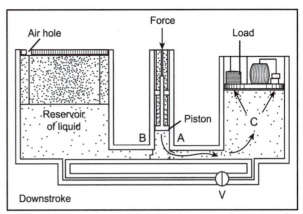

Figure 1-41. Hydraulic lift. A and B are valves. C is the hydraulic pressure to raise the load.

If air has been compressed, its properties will become more like that of an incompressible fluid. However, it still maintains some compressibility. A pneumatic device allows the air in a cylinder to be compressed by a moving piston followed by an increasing pressure within the cylinder. As the pressure is increased, the motion of the piston is opposed, and the compressed air tends to force the piston back in the opposite direction. Pneumatic devices, including pneumatic exercise machines, are based upon this principle.

Mass

Matter is anything that occupies space. The quantity or amount of matter is its mass. The mass of an object depends upon the volume and density of that object. An object has the same mass whether it is on the earth, on the moon, or traveling in a spaceship. Mass can also be considered to be resistance to linear motion. The greater the mass of an object, the more force is needed to either accelerate or decelerate the object. Mass is measured in kilograms or slugs.

When dealing with the mass of an object, the concept of center of mass is important. The center of mass is that point at the exact center of the object's mass (Figure 1-42). Often, this point is called the object's center of gravity. The force acting on the entire mass of a rigid object may be considered to act as a single force vector through the center of mass. This single vector represents the sum of many parallel forces distributed throughout the object. In the case of a symmetrical object, such as a cylinder or square block, the center of mass is also the geometric center of the object (see Figure 1-42). However, if the object is asymmetrical such as the limbs of the body, the center of mass is near the larger and heavier end (Figure 1-43). The center of mass of the entire body of the average person standing in the anatomical position is located within the pelvis (see Figure 1-43). It is generally higher in men than in women. Babies have their center of mass located in their trunk. The center of mass of the body changes as the individual moves and the body segments change position. Adding a weight, cast, or brace to the body or body part or having an amputation alters the mass and the center of mass of the individual. Methods to determine the center of mass of an object are presented in Chapter 7.

Moment of Inertia

The moment of inertia (I) in rotatory motion is analogous to mass in linear motion. The moment of inertia offers resistance to change in rotatory motion. Its value depends upon the

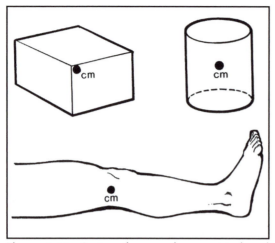

Figure 1-42. Center of mass of symmetrical and asymmetrical objects.

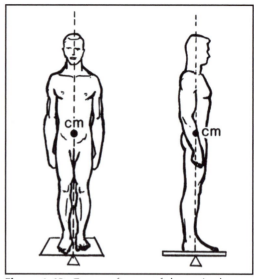

Figure 1-43. Center of mass of the entire human body.

mass of the object and the manner in which the mass is distributed. Consider that an object is composed of many small particles with each having a mass and a perpendicular distance from the center of rotation. Each particle (m) is located at a distance (r) from the center of rotation and contributes a resistance to the rotatory motion by the value of mr^2. The total moment of inertia is the sum of all of these particles (Figure 1-44), or

$$I = \Sigma mr^2$$

The moment of inertia for one point of mass would be $I = mr^2$ (Figure 1-45).

The moment of inertia of an object changes if the object is rotated around a different axis because the radius (r) of each particle will change (Figure 1-46). The axis of rotation must be specified in order for the moment of inertia to be meaningful. The radius of gyration in rotatory motion is analogous to the center of mass in linear motion. It is the location (k) in which the sum of masses of all particles is located without changing the value of the moment of inertia, or

$$I_{cm} = mk^2$$

The equation $I_{cm} = \Sigma mr^2$ is for the moment of inertia at the center of mass. When determining the effect of inertia on the body, the moment of inertia must be related to the axis of rotation at the joint. In this situation, the parallel axis theorem (Figure 1-47) is used. The moment of inertia around an axis parallel to the axis through the center of mass can be calculated as follows, where r_d is the distance of the center of gravity to the axis:

$$I_o = \Sigma mr^2 + mr_d^2$$

WORK

Work is defined as a force that causes displacement of an object (Figures 1-48 and 1-49). The magnitude of work (W) can be calculated using the magnitude of the force applied to move the object (F) times the magnitude of the displacement in the direction of the force, or the distance the object is moved (s). Thus, we have the equation for linear work as follows:

$$W = F \times s$$

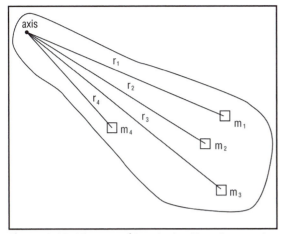

Figure 1-44. Moment of Inertia. $I = \Sigma m_1 r_1^2 + m_2 r_2^2 + m_3 r_3^2 + \ldots$

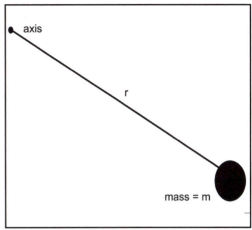

Figure 1-45. Moment of Inertia for a point of mass. $I = mr^2$

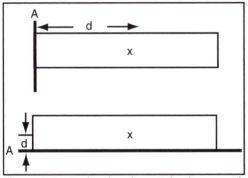

Figure 1-46. Radii of each particle change with the change in axis of a rotating object.

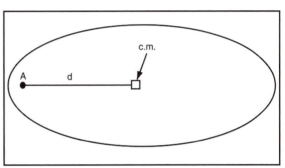

Figure 1-47. The parallel axis theorem. $I = \Sigma mr^2_{cm} + mr^2$.

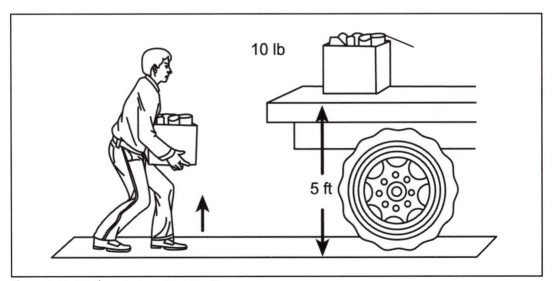

Figure 1-48. Work against gravity. W = Fs.

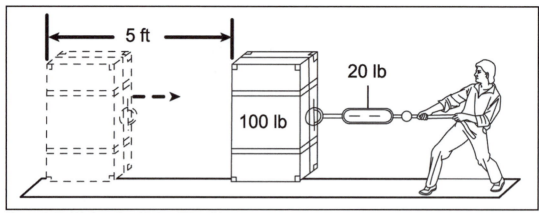

Figure 1-49. Work against friction. W = μNs.

If the force is acting at an angle to the direction of movement (Figure 1-50), then the force component acting in the direction of displacement is used, and the equation would be

$$W = F(\cos\Theta) \times s.$$
$$\text{Because } F = ma, \text{ then}$$
$$W = mas, \text{ or } W = ma(\cos\Theta) \times s$$

Work is done as an object is moved around an axis (Figure 1-51). The magnitude for such rotatory work is calculated using the torque applied to move a lever (T) times the magnitude of the angular displacement of the lever (Θ), or

$$W = T \times \Theta.$$
$$\text{Because } T = I\alpha \text{ and } I = mr^2, \text{ then}$$
$$W = mr^2\alpha\Theta$$

Work causes the transfer of energy from one object to another object. The units of work and energy are foot-pound (ft • lb), and Newton meter (N • m), or Joule (J).

EFFICIENCY

The efficiency of a machine, including the human machine, is related to the work that is done. The efficiency is usually presented as a percentage of the amount of work output divided by the work input multiplied by 100, or

$$\% \text{ Efficiency} = \left(\frac{\text{Work output}}{\text{Work input}}\right) \times 100$$

ENERGY

Energy is the capacity to do work or the ability to apply a force and move an object through a distance. Two forms of mechanical energy are potential energy and kinetic energy. The ability to do work because of the position of the object is called potential energy (PE). An object has stored energy because of its height or deformation. The formula for determining the potential energy of an object because of its height is

$$PE = mgh$$

Potential energy related to deformation is calculated by the formula as follows:

$$PE = \frac{1}{2}ks$$

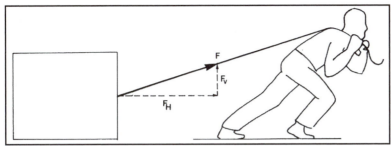

Figure 1-50. Frictional force acting at an angle. $W = F_f(\cos\theta)s$.

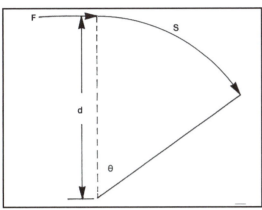

Figure 1-51. Work during angular motion. $W = (F \times d \times \theta)$, or $W = T\theta$.

Force acting on an object can perform work on the object by lifting it, deforming it, lowering it in a liquid, or changing its location in an electromagnetic field. In such situations, the object contains stored or potential energy because of its height, deformation, location in a fluid, or location in an electromagnetic field and will return the energy when the acting force is released.

The force acting on the object in this situation is considered to be a conservative force. In some situations, potential energy is not imparted to the object as work is performed on it. The energy from the work done is transferred from mechanical energy to non-recoverable heat and sound energy. The forces opposing the work being done are called non-conservative or dissipative forces. Examples of non-conservative forces are friction, viscoelastic materials, water and air resistance, and eddy currents from electromagnetic forces.

A moving object possesses energy because force must be applied to stop the object. The magnitude of energy of the moving object depends upon its mass and velocity. The mechanical energy of a moving object is called kinetic energy (KE) and is equal to one-half times its mass and velocity squared, or

$$KE = \tfrac{1}{2}mv^2$$

Potential energy and kinetic energy are shown to be related by the law of conservation of energy. This law states that energy can be neither created nor destroyed, but may be transformed from one form to another. If the small amount of heat and sound energy are disregarded, the sum of the potential energy and kinetic energy equals the total energy (TE).

$$TE = PE + KE$$

Because the total energy remains constant, when the potential energy decreases, the kinetic energy will increase and vice versa (Figures 1-52 and 1-53). However, to be complete, the total energy of an object at any time is the total of the potential energy, the kinetic energy, and the dissipated heat and sound energy.

$$TE = PE + KE + \text{heat} + \text{sound}$$

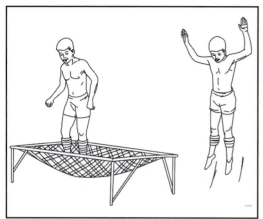

Figure 1-52. Jumping on a trampoline demonstrates change in potential and kinetic energy. Potential energy at the height of the jump and when the trampoline is fully stretched.

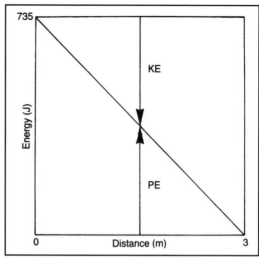

Figure 1-53. Graph of the relative values of potential and kinetic energy related to total energy.

POWER

Power is the rate of doing work or the rate of change of energy. Average power is the quantity of work done over a specific period of time. Power is calculated by the equations as follows:

$$\text{linear} \qquad P = \frac{W}{t} \text{ or } P = \frac{(F \times s)}{t}$$

$$\text{rotatory} \qquad P = \frac{W}{t} \text{ or } P = \frac{(T \times \Theta)}{t}$$

The units of power are foot-pound per second (ft • lb/sec), or horsepower (hp) and Joule per second (J/sec), or Watt (W). The relationship for these units is 1 hp = 550 ft • lb/sec = 746 W. Energy, work, and power will be covered in more detail in Chapter 6.

Newton's Laws of Motion

Newton's Laws of Motion (Table 1-2) have been presented separately earlier in the chapter. Now, they are stated and described to illustrate their relationship.

The first law is considered the law of inertia. This law has 3 parts:

1. An object at rest tends to remain at rest unless acted upon by an outside force.
2. An object in motion tends to remain in motion at a constant velocity unless acted upon by an outside force.
3. An object in motion tends to move in a straight line unless acted upon by an outside force.

The law of inertia is present everywhere. A box resting on a table does not move unless a force is applied to it. A fluid will remain in a pail as the pail is swung in a vertical circle (Figure 1-54). Mud flies in a straight line from a spinning tire (Figure 1-55). A racetrack or sled course must be banked on the curves to keep the vehicle on the track (Figure 1-56).

Newton's Second Law of Motion is the law of acceleration. This law is an extension of the first law of motion. It states that the acceleration (change in velocity or change in direction) of an object is directly proportional to the outside force acting on the object and inversely proportional

TABLE 1-2

Newton's Laws of Motion

- Inertia
- Acceleration ($a = \frac{F}{m}$)
- Reaction (Action = Reaction)

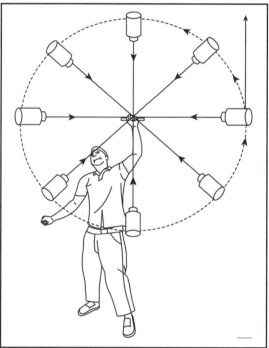

Figure 1-54. Inertia keeping fluid in a pail as the pail swings in a vertical circle.

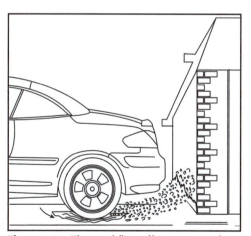

Figure 1-55. The mud flies off at a tangent from a rapidly spinning wheel.

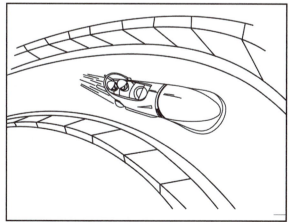

Figure 1-56. A sled needs banked curves to keep it on the track.

to the mass of the object. Accelerating a weight on a pulley system (Figure 1-57) is an example of this law. A large tackle on a football team is very difficult to move (accelerate) because of his large mass. A large running back is very difficult to stop (decelerate) because of his large mass and speed. A greater amount of force is needed to accelerate a bowling ball than a softball.

The law of reaction is Newton's Third Law. It states that for every action or force that is applied to an object, the object responds with an equal and opposite reaction. If you push against an object, it will push back against you with equal force in a direction exactly opposite to that of your push (Figure 1-58). If the object begins to move, the second law of motion becomes involved (Figure 1-59).

These laws will be considered throughout the text. The reader can think of many instances in which these laws apply. The first 2 laws are well-illustrated in normal walking. The lower limb must swing forward forcibly by action of the hip flexor muscles so that the foot may be placed ahead of the body as the center of mass travels forward. The leg swing is ballistic or thrust movement that, once begun, continues without further muscle effort. The swinging limb must then be stopped or decelerate in a controlled fashion by the hip extensors so that the heel can be brought to the ground at the proper time and place. Gravity is also a force in the acceleration of the limb at the beginning of the swing and in deceleration at the end of the swing. This swinging action of the limb in walking is like that of a damped pendulum that is forcibly accelerated and once started must be forcibly stopped. Without muscle forces, the limb would remain at rest or continue in motion beyond the proper point, making smooth walking impossible. The control of the arm swing by muscles in fast walking and running is another example of muscle activity used to overcome inertia of a body segment.

A body that is stationary or moving at a constant speed is moving in a state of equilibrium. A force must be applied to change this state. In case of a moving object, forces that help to slow down and stop this motion include 1) friction between the object and supporting surface and 2) air resistance. A patient being moved in a wheelchair may be thrown forward if the wheels suddenly catch on a door sill, or the patient's trunk is forced against the back of the chair when someone gives the chair an unexpected shove from behind. We have all had this experience while riding in an automobile when the driver suddenly applies the brake or the accelerator. Inertia causes an object to resist being set in motion or, if moving, to resist being slowed down or stopped. The inertia of an object is proportional to its weight. If an aide attempts to push a very heavy patient on a gurney, he has difficulty not only getting started but also stopping the motion at the end of the trip. Transporting a child would entail less resistance to starting and stopping. Likewise, an amputee needs to overcome less inertia in the control of the remaining portion of a limb than in control of the uninvolved limb. On the other hand, a limb in a cast or brace requires more than normal energy to control. The amount of decrease or increase of inertia is directly proportional to the change in mass. This is an important factor in energy expenditure and fatigue. Compare your own arm swing in walking when your hands are free with your swing when you are carrying a briefcase or handbag in your hand.

An example of the effect of inertia frequently seen in the clinic is the trauma sustained by the cervical spine in so-called whiplash injuries, or acute traumatic cervical syndrome (see Figure 1-25). Because the car in such accidents is usually bumped from the rear, the rider's head is first snapped into extension. This is because it attempts to remain at rest while the trunk is moved violently forward. The head is then thrown into a flexed position as the trunk comes to rest. In this way, the delicate structures on both the anterior and posterior aspects of the neck may be damaged. Brain damage in football injuries and other contact sports is also a similar type and is caused by the inertia of the brain.

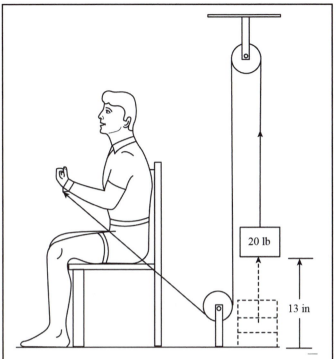

Figure 1-57. Accelerating a weight on a pulley systems requires more force than holding the weight.

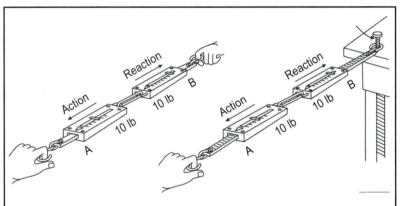

Figure 1-58. Action-reaction.

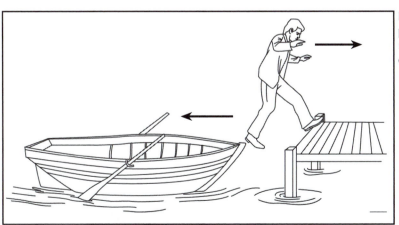

Figure 1-59. The boat is pushed backward as the man jumps forward because of reaction force.

Newton's Third Law regarding equal and opposite forces is illustrated by the usual floor or ground reaction in standing and walking. The supporting surface pushes upward against the sole of the foot with the same amount of force and along the same line of action as the downward force of the foot (see Figure 1-10). In locomotion, the character of the surface may be such that it fails to provide a counterforce to the foot and makes progress difficult and tiring as one walks on soft sand and gravel. Thin ice may supply the necessary equal and opposite reaction for a small boy, while his older brother will break through the surface. If a crutch or a cane is placed on the floor in a vertical position, it is very stable since the floor pushes vertically upward in return. However, if a crutch is placed far out to the side at an angle to the body, the action line of the reaction force is at a corresponding angle with the vertical, and the crutch is more likely to slip. A person taking long strides is more apt to slide forward when the heel strikes a slippery floor than one who takes shorter steps with the foot coming down in a more vertical angle. Horizontal force, such as that which accompanies the push off in walking, must be opposed by an equal and opposite force so that the foot is stable and progression can take place. Friction between the sole of the foot and the ground normally supplies the necessary counterforce. Lack of friction, as on a slippery surface, will make normal walking difficult or impossible. In our daily life, all posture and movement is constantly influenced by the surface that supports us. We may not be conscious of this because, through experience, our adjustments have become largely automatic. Contrast your movement in stepping off a curb into the street with stepping into a small canoe on a lake. Unfamiliar or unstable supporting surfaces require control of movement on a conscious level. A patient with paraplegia may face frustration and possible injury if he or she attempts to get into a bed that has freely rolling casters or forgets to lock the wheelchair or back it against a wall before sitting down in it. He or she cannot execute the movement successfully unless an adequate counterforce from a stable bed or chair is provided.

Activities

1. Give examples of the biomechanics that you have seen in clinical and everyday use.
2. Define and give an example of each of the following terms:

acceleration	extensibility	motor unit
biomechanics	force	Newton's First Law
buoyancy	four characteristics of force	Newton's Second Law
center of gravity	friction	Newton's Third Law
center of mass	Hooke's Law	non-conservative force
concentric	hydraulics	parallel axis theorem
conservation of energy	inertia	Pascal's Law
conservative force	isometric	pneumatics
contractility	isotonic	potential energy
deceleration	joint reaction force	power
eccentric	kinetic energy	pressure
Eddy currents	load	scalar
elasticity	mass	strength
energy	matter	torque
excitability	moment of inertia	vector

3. Draw an example of force, labeling its 4 characteristics.
   a. A client lying prone with the knee flexed 30 degrees and cuff weight on the ankle.

b. A client standing with the upper limb abducted 90 degrees and dumbbell or elastic band in the hand.

c. A client sidelying with the hip abducted 20 degrees and a cuff weight on the ankle.

d. A client standing flexed at the hips lifting a box.

e. A client sitting with the elbow flexed 90 degrees and dumbbell, elastic band, pulley cord, or variable resistance handle in his hand.

f. A client standing performing heel raises.

g. The elbow extensors as an individual pushes a large box along the floor.

h. An individual walking at heel contact.

i. An individual walking during swing phase just prior to heel contact.

j. Someone standing in a pool with paddles on his hands adducting the arms.

4. Give an example for each of the 8 types of force.

5. Differentiate among isometric, concentric, and eccentric contractions.

6. Contrast the 2 definitions of strength.

7. Discuss the concept of pressure related to prevention of injury, treatment techniques, and everyday activities.

8. Compare hydraulics and pneumatics and provide examples of each.

9. Compare the concepts of mass and moment of inertia, and provide examples of each.

10. Relate the concepts of energy, work, and power.

11. Give an example of exercise for each type of force presented and briefly describe it. Explain.

12. State Newton's 3 laws and give clinical examples of each.

13. Explain how the types of force presented can or cannot provide exercise resistance in a space station.

14. Describe the relationships within each equation in Table 1-3.

TABLE 1-3

Equations

$F = ma$	$I = \sum mr^2 + mr_d^2$
$a = \frac{F}{m}$	$W = Fs$
$F_g = \frac{Gm_1 m_2}{r^2}$	$W = T\Theta$
$F = -kl$	$PE = mgh$
$F_s = \mu N$	$PE = \frac{1}{2}ks$
$F = W - B$	$KE = \frac{1}{2}mv^2$
$T = F_d$	$KE = \frac{1}{2}I\omega^2$
$P = \frac{F}{A}$	$TE = PE + KE$
$I = \sum mr^2$	$P = \frac{W}{t}$

Suggested Reading List

Benzel EC. The essentials of spine biomechanics for the general neurosurgeon. *Clin Neurosurg.* 2003;50:86-177.

Bluestein D, Javaheri A. Pressure ulcers: prevention, evaluation, and management. *Am Fam Physician.* 2008;78(10):1186-1194.

Chan KM, Fong DT, Hong Y, Yung PS, Lui PP. Orthopaedic sport biomechanics—a new paradigm. *Clin Biomech (Bristol, Avon).* 2008;23(suppl 1):S21-S30.

Chao EY. Orthopaedic biomechanics. The past, present and future. *Int Orthop.* 1996;20(4):239-243.

Chleboun GS, Patel TJ, Lieber RL. Skeletal muscle architecture and fiber-type distribution with the multiple bellies of the mouse extensor digitorum longus muscle. *Acta Anat (Basel).* 1997;159(2-3):147-155.

Crenshaw RP, Vistnes LM. A decade of pressure sore research: 1977-1987. *J Rehabil Res Dev.* 1989;26(1):63-74.

Cress NM, Peters KS, Chandler JM. Eccentric and concentric force-velocity relationships of the quadriceps femoris muscle. *J Orthop Sports Phys Ther.* 1992;16(2):82-86.

Daniel RK, Priest DL, Wheatley DC. Etiologic factors in pressure sores: an experimental model. *Arch Phys Med Rehabil.* 1981;62(10):492-498.

Drillis R, Contini R, Bluestein M. Body segment parameters; a survey of measurement techniques. *Artif Limbs.* 1964;25:44-66.

Gordon AM, Huxley AF, Julian FJ. The variation in isometric tension with sarcomere length in vertebrate muscle fibers. *J Physiol.* 1966;184(1):170-192.

Hatze H. A mathematical model for the computational determination of parameter values of anthropomorphic segments. *J Biomech.* 1980;13(10):833-843.

Herbert RD, Gandevia SC. Changes in pennation with joint angle and muscle torque: in vivo measurements in human brachialis muscle. *J Physiol.* 1995;484(Pt 2):523-532.

Herzog W, Lee EJ, Rassier DE. Residual force enhancement in skeletal muscle. *J Physiol.* 2006;574 (Pt 3):635-642.

Kawakami Y, Abe T, Fukunaga T. Muscle-fiber pennation angles are greater in hypertrophied than in normal muscles. *J Appl Physiol.* 1993;74(6):2740-2744.

Kawakami Y, Fukunaga T. New insights into in vivo human skeletal muscle function. *Exerc Sport Sci Rev.* 2006;34(1):16-21.

Kellis E, Baltzopoulis V. Muscle activation differences between eccentric and concentric isokinetic exercise. *Med Sci Sports Exerc.* 1998;30(11):1616-1623.

Komi PV. Measurement of the force-velocity relationship in human muscle under concentric and eccentric contractions. In Cerquiglini S, Venerando S, Wartenweiler J, eds. *Biomechanics III.* Baltimore, MD: University Park Press; 1973:224-229.

Latash ML, Zatsiorsky VM. *Classics in Movement Science.* Champaign, IL: Human Kinetics; 2001.

Lieber RL. Skeletal muscle architecture: implications for muscle function and surgical tendon transfer. *J Hand Ther.* 1993;6(2):105-113.

Lieber RL, Bodine-Fowler SC. Skeletal muscle mechanics: implications for rehabilitation. *Phys Ther.* 1993;73(12):844-856.

Lieber RL, Fridén J. Clinical significance of skeletal muscle architecture. *Clin Orthop Relat Res.* 2001;(383):140-151.

Lieber RL, Fridén J. Functional and clinical significance of skeletal muscle architecture. *Muscle Nerve.* 2000;23(11):1647-1666.

Mademli L, Arampatzis A. Behaviour of the human gastrocnemius muscle architecture during submaximal isometric fatigue. *Eur J Appl Physiol.* 2005;94(5-6):611-617.

McInnes E, Bell-Syer SE, Dumville JC, Legood R, Cullum NA. Support surfaces for pressure ulcer prevention. *Cochrane Database Syst Rev.* 2008:CD001735.

Mohamed O, Perry J, Hislop H. Relationship between wire EMG activity, muscle length, and torque of the hamstrings. *Clin Biomech (Bristol, Avon)*. 2002;17(8):569-579.

Mow VC, Flatow EL, Ateshian GA. Biomechanics. In Buckwalter JA, Einhorn TA, Simon SR, eds. *Orthopaedic Basic Science: Biology and Biomechanics of the Musculoskeletal System*. 2nd ed. Rosemont, IL: American Academy of Orthopaedic Surgery; 2000:133-181.

Mow VC, Huiskes R. A brief history of science and orthopaedic biomechanics. In Mow VC, Huiskes R, eds. *Basic Orthopaedics Biomechanics and Mechano-Biology*. 3rd ed. Philadelphia, PA: Lippincott, Williams and Wilkins; 2005:1-27.

Mow VC, Huiskes R, eds. *Basic Orthopaedic Biomechanics and Mechano-Biology*. 3rd ed. Philadelphia, PA: Lippincott, Williams and Wilkins; 2005.

Neumann ES. Measurement of socket discomfort—Part I: Pressure sensation. *J Prosth Orthot*. 2001;13(4):99-110.

Reger SI, Ranganathan VK, Sahgal V. Support surface interface pressure, microenvironment, and the prevalence of pressure ulcers: an analysis of the literature. *Ostomy Wound Manage*. 2007;53(10):50-58.

Schachar R, Herzog W, Leonard TR. Force enhancement above the initial isometric force on the descending limb of the force-length relationship. *J Biomech*. 2002;35(10):1299-1306.

Singh M, Karpovich PV. Isotonic and isometric forces. *J Appl Physiol*. 1966;21(4):1435-1437.

Stotthart JP. Relationship between selected biomechanical parameters of static and dynamic performance. In Cerquiglini S, Venerando S, Wartenweiler J, eds. *Biomechanics III*. Baltimore, MD: University Park Press; 1973:210-217.

Swain ID, Bader DL. The measurement of interface pressure and its role in soft tissue breakdown. *J Tissue Viability*. 2002;12(4):132-134, 136-137, 140-146.

Then C, Menger J, Benderoth G, et al. Analysis of mechanical interaction between human gluteal soft tissue and body supports. *Technol Health Care*. 2008;16(1):61-76.

Ward SR, Eng CM, Smallwood LH, Lieber RL. Are current measurements of lower extremity muscle architecture accurate? *Clin Orthop Relat Res*. 2009;467(4):1074-1082.

Ward SR, Hentzen ER, Smallwood LH, et al. Rotator cuff muscle architecture: implications for glenohumeral stability. *Clin Orthop Relat Res*. 2006;448:157-163.

Ward SR, Kim CW, Eng CM, et al. Architectural analysis and intraoperative measurements demonstrate the unique design of the multifidus muscle for lumbar spine stability. *J Bone Joint Surg Am*. 2009;91(1):176-185.

Wickiewicz TL, Roy RR, Powell PL, Perrine JJ, Edgerton VR. Muscle architecture and force-velocity relationships in humans. *J Appl Physiol*. 1984;57(2):435-443.

Wilcox RK. An introduction to basic mechanics. *Current Orthopaedics*. 2006;20:1-8.

Woo SL, Thomas M, Chan Saw SS. Contribution of biomechanics, orthopaedics and rehabilitation: the past, present, and future. *Surgeon*. 2004;2(3):125-136.

Zajac FE. How musculotendon architecture and joint geometry affect the capacity of muscles to move and exert force on objects: a review with application to arm and forearm tendon transfer design. *J Hand Surg Am*. 1992;17(5):799-804.

Zatsiorsky V, Seluyanov V. The mass and inertial characteristics of the main segments of the human body. In Matsui HK, ed. *Biomechanics VIII-B*. Champaign, IL: Human Kinetics; 1983:1152-1159.

chapter **2**

Strength of Materials

Objectives

1. Define basic terms.
2. Differentiate between stress and strain.
3. Differentiate and give examples of the 3 principle stresses.
4. Draw and label a "typical" stress-strain or load-strain curve.
5. Explain the effect and locate the stresses during the loading of an object.
6. Analyze and describe the effects of force on growth.
7. Explain examples of strength of materials in the clinic.
8. Differentiate among resilience, damping, and toughness.
9. Differentiate between fatigue and creep.
10. Give examples of strength of materials in the medical, rehabilitation, sports medicine, and exercise science fields.

Loading

Knowledge of the behavior of biological materials and biomaterials is important for the practitioners who deal with the human body. Biological materials are often affected by forces external to the material. Research continues to reveal the responses of loads on the mechanical characteristics of bone, cartilage, vertebral discs, menisci, tendons, and ligaments. Recent studies have been investigating the responses of these structures at the cellular level to determine cell-mediated remodeling events that occur when loads are applied.

Knowledge of the effect of loads on biomaterials provides an understanding for the repair or replacement of biological tissues. A newly developed approach to studying biomaterials is biomimetrics. This approach involves imitating living tissues with nonliving materials. The use of biomaterials has advanced from inert materials to materials that assist with regeneration.

As a load is imposed upon the material, the load tends to deform (change in size or shape) the material. In turn, the material tends to resist this deformation. The amount of deformation depends upon the magnitude of the load and the ability of the material to resist the deformation. The ability of the material to resist deformation is often referred to as the strength of the material.

LeVeau BF.
Biomechanics of Human Motion: Basics and Beyond for the Health Professions (pp 35-54).
© 2011 SLACK Incorporated

Figure 2-1. The 3 principle stresses or strains.

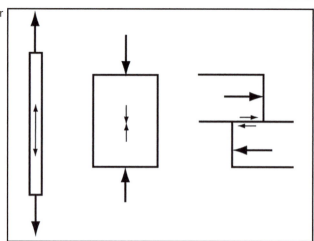

As the load acts on the material and the material tends to resist, a change in size and shape may occur. This change can often be determined by measuring the change in length of the object or the change in an angle within the object. This change in dimensions is called strain. Because strain is the change in length divided by the original length $(S = \frac{\Delta l}{l})$, strain has no dimensions. The property of a material to resist the deformation caused by forces acting on it is called mechanical stress. The units for stress are force per unit area.

THREE PRINCIPAL STRAINS AND STRESSES

Three principal strains and stresses exist (Figure 2-1). Tension occurs when 2 or more external forces act on the material along the same line of application (collinear) in opposite directions away from each other. The material tends to be pulled apart (Figure 2-2). Compression occurs when 2 or more forces act on the material along the same line of application in opposite directions directed toward each other (Figure 2-3). In this case, the material tends to be pressed together. The third strain or stress is shearing. Shearing occurs when 2 or more parallel but non-collinear forces pointed in opposite directions act on the material (Figure 2-4). The adjacent surfaces of the material tend to slide past each other.

These 3 stresses may arise within the body by axial (direct or linear) loading or by loads acting at a distance, such as bending or torsion. Axial, bending, and torsion loading may occur alone or in some combination. In all instances, tension, compression, and shear occur in some degree when the material is loaded. The resulting stress and strain are related to the force components applied to the material.

AXIAL LOADS

Loading along the axis of an object is referred to as axial loading. An object such as an intervertebral disc (Figure 2-5) that is loaded by collinear (along the same line of application) forces acting toward each other will have compressive stress. The height of the disc will tend to decrease, and the disc will get wider. The widening of the disc illustrates that tension stresses are also developed perpendicular to the line of application of the loads. Shear stresses will be produced at angles of 45 degrees to the loads. Similarly, a ligament, tendon, muscle, or other soft tissue that is stretched by tension-producing loads will become narrower. This narrowing of the tissue shows that compression stress is also involved. Shear stresses will also be developed at 45 degrees to the load in this situation.

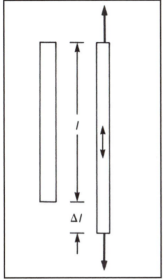

Figure 2-2. Tension strain.

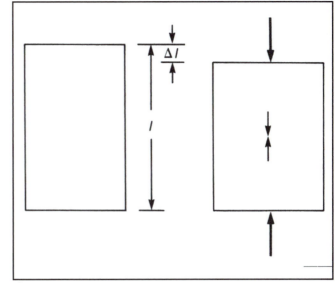

Figure 2-3. Compression strain.

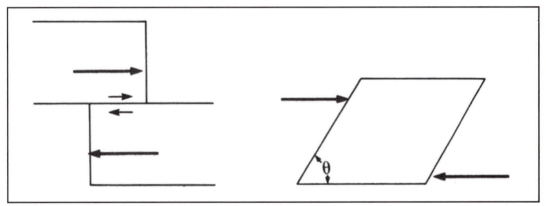

Figure 2-4. Shearing strain.

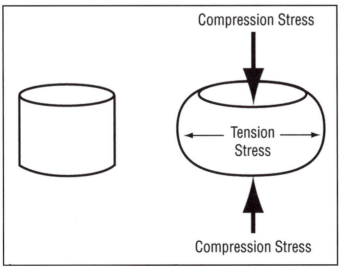

Figure 2-5. Axial loading (compression strain on the object with tension strain on the vertical edges).

Figure 2-6. Bending strain from loading of end-supported beam with loads at the end supports and a load in the opposite direction between the supports (3-point principle). Compression occurs in the concave area, tension in the convex area, and shear parallel and perpendicular to the loads.

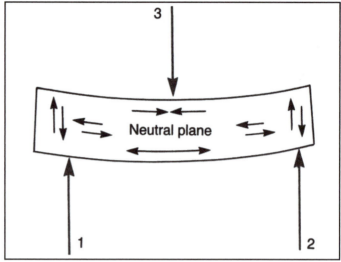

Bending Loads

Bending of an object occurs when forces or force components act in a coplanar manner but are not collinear. These forces lie in the same plane but do not have the same line of application or point of application.

A beam that is supported at both ends with a load (or loads) between the ends demonstrates a bending situation (Figure 2-6). The load can be a gravitational force that causes contact forces to be developed at the supporting ends. The greater the gravitational force, the greater the supporting contact forces will be. These forces tend to cause the beam to bend or develop a curvature. Compression stress will arise in the concave (top) side of the beam, and tension stress develops in the convex (bottom) side of the beam. Shearing stresses in a homogenous material are present within the beam perpendicular and parallel to the forces. The amount of bending and stress depend upon the magnitude and the location of the forces. Greater bending and related stresses are developed if the magnitude of the forces is increased or if the distance between the supporting forces is increased. These loading systems are often referred to as the 3-point and 4-point bending systems used by many braces, casts, and splints (Figures 2-7 and 2-8).

Figure 2-9 illustrates an example of a loaded beam in the body as a weight-bearing foot. As an individual stands, the heel and the ball of the foot are the supporting surfaces. The gravitational force is the weight of the body. Tension stresses develop in the ligaments and plantar fascia along the plantar surface of the foot. Compression stresses act between the bones of the foot. Shearing will occur parallel to the surfaces of the bones. Because the foot is not a homogenous material, these lines of stress are not exactly parallel or perpendicular to the forces. Numerous other examples exist within and in relation to the human body.

An eccentrically loaded beam is considered to be a cantilever. In the simplest situation, a horizontal beam is supported and anchored at one end, while the other free end is loaded like a diving board (Figure 2-10A). The loaded beam tends to bend, producing stresses and strains in the beam (Figure 2-10B). Tension stress and strain will occur in the upper convex side of the beam. Compression stress and strain will occur in the lower concave side of the beam. Shearing stress and strain will be perpendicular and parallel to the applied forces. The magnitude of the stress and resulting strain depends upon the magnitude of the load and the location of the point of application of the load on the beam. As with the beam, the greater the magnitude or the greater the distance of the load from the supported end, the greater the amount of bending.

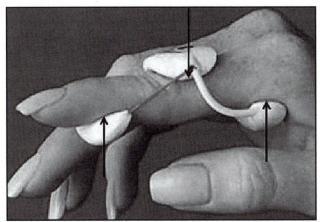

Figure 2-7. The 3-point principle used by the LMB Spring Finger Extension Splint. Reprinted with permission from Patterson Medical/Sammons Preston, Bolingbrook, IL.

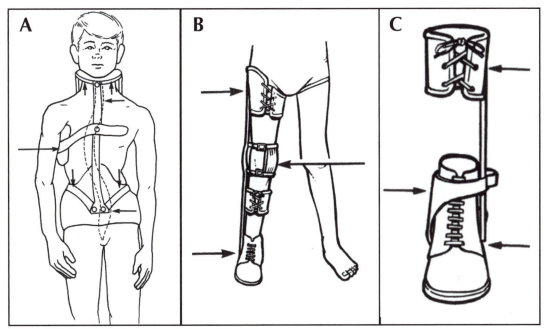

Figure 2-8. Braces using the 3-point principle.

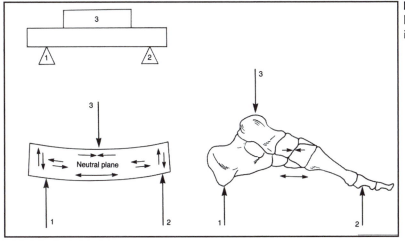

Figure 2-9. The foot as a loaded beam demonstrating the 3-point principle.

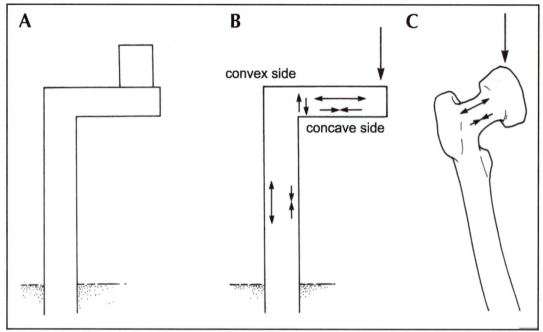

Figure 2-10. Eccentrically loaded beam.

In the human body, the proximal end of the femur represents an eccentrically loaded cantilever (Figure 2-10C). The body weight loads the head of the femur so that the neck of the femur tends to bend. Tension stress is developed in the upper part of the femoral neck. Compression stress is produced in the lower aspect of the femoral neck. Shearing occurs along the epiphyseal plate. Femoral neck fractures and slipping of the epiphysis are related to these stresses. Other examples occur within and in contact with the human body, including the diving board, a baseball bat, and some splint situations.

Torsion Loads

When a rod or shaft is loaded so that it will twist around its long axis, torsion is developed (Figure 2-11). Forces on one end of the rod tend to rotate it clockwise, and forces on the other end of the rod tend to rotate it counterclockwise. When torsion occurs, tension, compression, and shearing stresses and strains are produced. Tension and compression stresses are located along spiraling lines along the length of the rod. Shearing stresses are perpendicular and parallel to the rod. The magnitude of the stresses depends upon the magnitude of the applied loads and the location of the points of application from the long axis of the rod.

The force overcoming the friction resistance when removing a lid from a jar illustrates the perpendicular shearing stress of torsion (Figure 2-12). A spiral fracture of the tibia is an example of a bone failing because of torsion loading (see Figure 2-11C). The spiral fracture line indicates the failure of tension stress to resist the breaking of the bone. A spiral fracture of the humerus can also occur (Figure 2-13). The muscle forces of the rotator cuff hold the proximal end of the humerus, while the inertial forces of the forearm and hand act on the distal end of the limb. Occasionally, splints are placed on the legs of children in an attempt to correct torsional growth deformities.

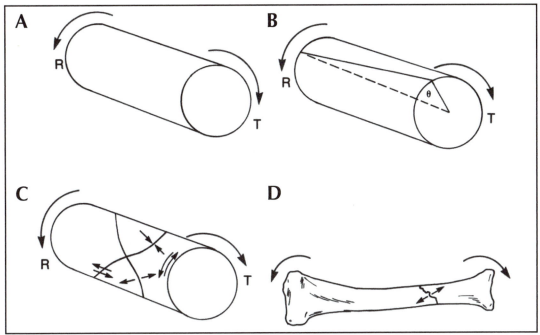

Figure 2-11. Torsion load (spiral fracture of the tibia).

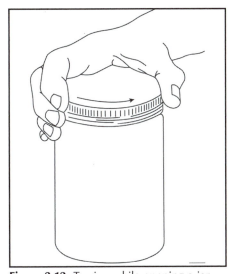

Figure 2-12. Torsion while opening a jar.

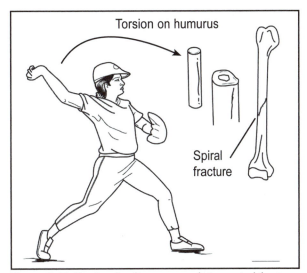

Figure 2-13. Torsion loading can result in a spiral fracture.

Rheological Properties

ELASTICITY

As presented in Chapter 1, some materials demonstrate the property of elasticity. That is, they have the capacity to return immediately to their original size and shape once they have been deformed. The relationship between a load and deformation known as Hooke's Law is a straight line in a purely elastic material. Such a material returns all of the energy applied to it. A spring, rubber ball, and an elastic resistance band are examples of this behavior.

VISCOSITY

A viscous material does not deform instantaneously when a load is applied and does not return immediately to its original size and shape when the load is removed. The stress within the material will occur, but the strain is delayed. The stress within a viscous material depends upon the rate of loading. The greater the rate of loading (the faster the load is applied), the greater the stress developed. A constant rate of loading produces a constant stress. A viscoelastic material deforms slowly in a nonlinear fashion. When the load is removed, the material will slowly and nonlinearly return toward its original size and shape. Some energy is lost in the form of heat because of the viscous reaction. The property of viscoelasticity combines the elastic reaction of a spring with a dashpot or syringe type of reaction similar to the damper on a screen door. The dashpot provides a damping effect that resists the rapid rate of change in length of a tissue. This damping effect is similar to what happens when a fluid is forced through a syringe (Figure 2-14). The small opening at the end of a syringe retards the rapid rate of plunger motion. Screen door closers and some exercise devices operate on this principle. The elastic property allows deformation of the tissue in direct proportion to the force applied and an immediate return to its original size and shape when the force is released. The combined viscoelastic response of the tissue allows for a slow movement of the material and return of the material to its original size and shape. The actions of a viscoelastic material can be illustrated by a model having a spring and dashpot connected in series. Most biological materials demonstrate viscoelastic behavior.

When muscles (including connective tissue) are stretched, they react in a manner similar to that of other materials with viscoelastic properties. Some other body tissues have elastin and collagen fibers, which provides for a viscoelastic response when they are stretched by a force. When the force is released, the tissue rebounds to its previous shape. The viscoelastic property of the muscle aids in the smooth control of human movement and may protect the muscle from injury.

PLASTICITY

Unlike an elastic material, a material displaying plastic behavior does not completely return to its original size and shape. A material that demonstrates the property of plasticity retains some of its change in size or shape when the deforming load is removed. An elastic material may exhibit plastic behavior if the material is strained beyond its elastic limit. The behavior of such a material can be demonstrated by the stress-strain diagram (Figure 2-15).

Stress-Strain Relationship

The relationship between stress and strain in an elastic material reveals a straight line (see Figure 2-15). This relationship is known as Hooke's Law. The basis of the law is that as a load is applied to the material, the strain or deformation is directly proportional to the stress developed within the material. As a load is applied to a material, the material begins to deform. The deformation depends upon the magnitude of the applied load and the ability of the material to resist the load. A stiff material can tolerate a large load with little deformation, while a less stiff material responds with a large deformation to low loads (Figure 2-16). A stiff material will have a steep slope on the stress-strain curve, while a less stiff material will have a less steep slope. The slope of the curve is determined by the ratio of stress (σ) to strain (ε). This ratio defines the modulus of elasticity (E), or Young's modulus ($E = \frac{\sigma}{\varepsilon}$). The higher the value for E, the stiffer the material. Steel and dry bone are stiff materials. A rubber band is less stiff. The proportional limit is the point on the diagram after which the strain is no longer proportional to the stress.

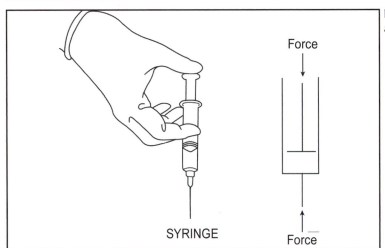

Figure 2-14. Damping occurs in a syringe.

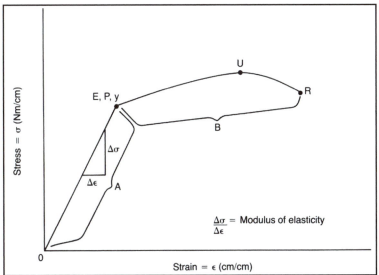

Figure 2-15. Stress-strain curve: E = elastic limit; P = proportional limit; y = yield point; U = ultimate point; R = rupture point; A = elastic range; B = plastic range; $\frac{\Delta\sigma}{\Delta\varepsilon}$ = modulus of elasticity.

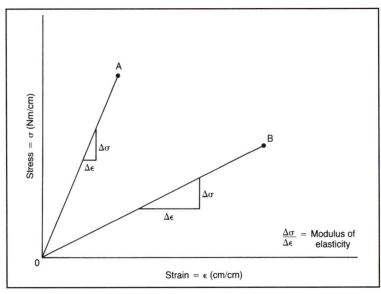

Figure 2-16. Representation of stiffness. Line A has a greater modulus of elasticity and is stiffer than line B.

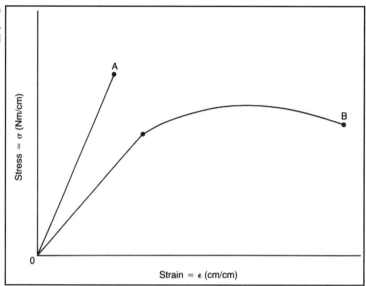

Figure 2-17. Representation of (A) brittle and (B) ductile materials. A brittle material has no or limited plastic deformation.

The elastic limit is at this same point or slightly beyond the proportional limit. This is the maximal stress that the material can take without permanent deformation. The region of the diagram extending from the origin to the elastic limit is called the elastic range. If the load is removed within this range, the material will return to its original size and shape. Beyond the elastic limit, the material is no longer elastic (inelastic).

At a point on the diagram (see Figure 2-15) following the elastic limit is a point in some materials called the yield point. At this point, the strain becomes much greater than the corresponding stress. After yielding is complete, the material regains some of its elastic capabilities, and further strain is accompanied by a corresponding stress. The highest point on the diagram is called the ultimate strength of the material. After this point, the strain continues with a decrease in the stress until rupture occurs. The region from the elastic limit to the point of rupture is called the plastic range.

A brittle material is one that has little or no plastic deformation. The rupture point is near the elastic limit. Chalk, glass, and dry bone are examples of a brittle material. A ductile material, in contrast, is a material that has a large plastic range. Ductility refers to the ability of a material to sustain a great amount of deformation before it ruptures. Aluminum and copper are good examples of ductile materials. Stress-strains curves for a brittle material and a ductile material are shown in Figure 2-17.

The work done by a load on a material is determined by the area under the stress-strain curve. As a material is loaded, the work done on the material increases the energy within the material. The area under the elastic region of the curve represents the stored strain energy of the material (Figure 2-18).

As the material is unloaded, this energy is generally recovered. If the strain has gone beyond the elastic limit, some of the energy will be transformed into the form of heat, and not all of the energy can be recovered. The resilience of a material is its ability to absorb and release energy (Figure 2-19). It is the ability to return to its original size and shape with vigor. A highly resilient material will rebound to its original size and shape with the same briskness as it was deformed with little or no energy given off as heat during loading and unloading. Damping is the characteristic that delays the return of a material to its original size and shape.

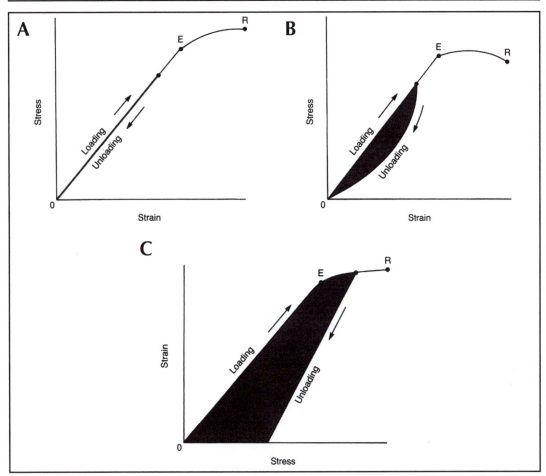

Figure 2-18. The area under the stress-strain curve represents stored strain energy of the material. Resilience and damping during loading and unloading; the shaded area represents energy lost. (A) Resilient material. (B) Energy lost in less resilient material. (C) Energy lost when loading takes a material into the plastic range.

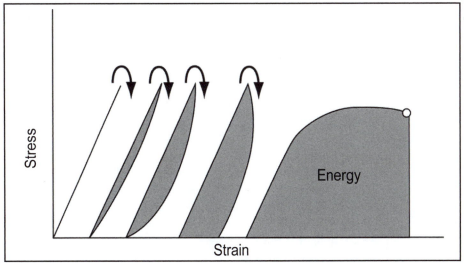

Figure 2-19. Resilience-Toughness. Comparison of resilient and tough materials. Tough materials absorb a large amount of energy before rupturing.

A material that demonstrates the property of damping has a loss of energy during loading and unloading. As a material undergoes cyclical loading, energy is changed to the form of heat. This form of energy dissipation is called hysteresis. The dissipated energy, the energy used to permanently deform a material, is determined by the area between the loading and unloading curves. If loading causes the strain to go into the plastic range, considerable energy may be dissipated as heat energy. The toughness of a material is the amount of work needed to rupture a material. As shown in Figure 2-19, a tough material absorbs a large amount of energy before it breaks.

A material may rupture because of mechanical fatigue, which is the failure of a material caused by repeated cyclic loading (Figure 2-20). The greater the magnitude of the load, the fewer cycles will be needed before rupture occurs. A lower load will require more cycles before the material breaks. The endurance limit of a material is the load at which an infinite number of cycles may occur without failure. A stress fracture is an example of the breaking of a bone caused by mechanical fatigue.

Another phenomenon that can cause a material to rupture is called creep. Creep occurs as material is continuously loaded for a prolonged time (Figure 2-21). The greater the load, the faster the material will deform toward failure. A very low load may not be sufficient to cause creep to occur. A phenomenon related to creep is stress relaxation. Stress relaxation occurs when a material is deformed by a load at a constant strain, and over a period of time the stress decreases (Figure 2-22). Traction, splinting, and serial casting may use the phenomena of creep and stress relaxation.

Effects of Loading Biological Tissue

Biological tissues are living materials and readily respond to the presence and absence of loads applied to them. Biomechanical factors play a major part in influencing the processes of tissue growth, development, maintenance, degeneration, and repair. The enhancement or deprivation of stresses within a tissue reacting to a load influence the tissue's structure and mechanical characteristics. For example, muscle becomes smaller and weaker when it is not used, but a muscle that is used becomes larger and stronger. Similar responses occur in other living tissues.

Loads can greatly modify the size, shape, and strength of bone, cartilage, ligaments, and tendons. The ability of bone to adapt by changing its size, shape, and internal structure depends upon the mechanical stresses established by the load. This ability is often referred to as Wolff's Law. Early in life, tissue differentiation and growth seems to follow loading of muscle contraction of the embryo and fetus and the muscular activity of the mother. Intrauterine bone loading of the fetus from movement and kicking against the uterus appears to be critical for normal fetal bone formation. Mechanical stresses are important for early skeletal development. The progression of infant and juvenile musculoskeletal deformities and their clinical management is related to mechanical forces. Bone density in children with cerebral palsy is greatly decreased, and fractures may occur with minimal trauma.

The type of loading has effects upon the type of tissues developed and the amount and direction of tissue growth. In general, large loads (within limits) increase the size and strength of tissues. Zero load or low loads lead to a decrease in the size and strength of the tissues. Weight-bearing activity (ie, walking/running) and muscle strengthening exercises can increase bone mass, direct trabecular growth, and retard tissue atrophy because these types of activities place loads on the body. Nonweight-bearing activities allow bone mass to decrease and ligaments to weaken.

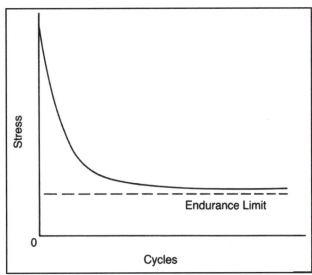

Figure 2-20. Mechanical fatigue: Relationship between stress at failure to number of cycles of loading. Endurance limit is level of stress below which an infinite number of cycles will not cause failure.

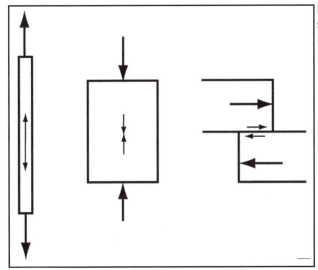

Figure 2-21. Creep phenomenon: Increasing strain occurring because of prolonged loading.

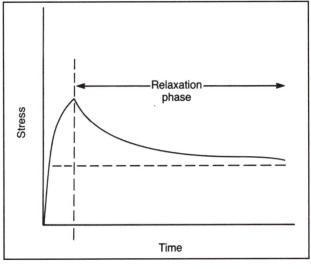

Figure 2-22. Stress relaxation: The stress on an object loaded under a constant strain is reduced with length of item loaded.

Many examples of the effect of loads on growth exist. Tennis players, both men and women, have greater bone cortex thickness of the upper limb on the playing side compared with the non-playing side. Disabled children who stand have more normally developed hips and femurs than those who do not stand. Individuals who take part in weight-training exercises have denser bones than individuals who do not weight train. Exercise has been shown to increase the strength of ligaments and tendons. Weight-bearing exercise and weight training can help retard loss of bone and soft tissue strength. Early passive motion following injury appears to increase the strength of damaged fibrous tissues and accelerate tissue healing. Studies, however, have also provided a warning about forces on tissues. Decreases in tissue mass and strength can occur during immobilization of a body or body part. Immobilization may be imposed by such situations as prolonged bed rest or casting of a limb. Most individuals readily notice the muscle atrophy that occurs; however, they rarely realize that other tissues have also been similarly affected. Bone, cartilage, ligaments, and tendons also tend to atrophy and lose strength. Bone mineral loss because of immobilization has been seen in patients with paralysis or fractures. Space travel may be limited because of loss of bone minerals brought about by weightlessness. Articular cartilage and ligaments deteriorate with immobilization. Sufficient loads are needed to retard or to eliminate tissue atrophy. Following prolonged immobilization, improvement in tissue strength with exercise will take a very long time.

Too much force or force applied too early after injury may cause increased damage. Prolonged loading may also have adverse effects on tissues. Constant loading may cause breakdown of the material by mechanical means of creep or by restricting blood flow and nutrition to the area. Early prolonged loading may create deformities of bone and cartilage, such as club foot or hip dysplasia. Such deformity problems must be corrected at an early age. The size, shape, and strength of tissues are determined by the characteristics of the loads applied to them. A clinician can influence what these force characteristics will be. The clinician must be cognizant of the magnitude of force necessary for the most efficient rehabilitation of the patient.

Biomaterials are used for internal implants. A material is selected for its specific use depending upon its mechanical, physical, and chemical properties. An attempt is made to choose specific material that most closely resembles the properties of the replaced tissue. Biomaterials are used for such items as joint replacements; endoskeletal fixation; bone graft substitutes; surgical sutures; synthetic grafts; dental materials; and artificial tendons, ligaments, and skin. The materials used include metals, ceramics and glass, polymers, natural materials, and composites. Many textbooks and journal articles have presented the details of the use of these materials within the body.

External orthotic and prosthetic materials are constantly being improved. Energy-absorbing prosthetic feet, ankle foot orthoses, computerized knee joints, prosthetic limb sockets, and various splints are examples of materials that are changing.

Activities

1. Compare the following:
   a. load, stress, and strain
   b. tension, compression, and shear
   c. axial, eccentric, bending, and torsional loading
   d. elastic, viscous, and viscoelastic
   e. brittle and ductile
   f. resilience, hysteresis, and toughness
   g. fatigue, creep, and stress relaxation

2. Draw and label a stress-strain curve for a brittle and ductile material.

3. Discuss the effect the rate of loading has on a material.

4. Provide examples and discuss the use of strength of materials and concepts in the body, in clinical use, and in everyday activities.

5. Define the following terms.

axial load	eccentric load	point of rupture
bending	elastic limit	proportional limit
brittle	elastic range	resilience
cantilever	elasticity	shear
collinear	endurance limit	stiff
compression	Hooke's Law	strain
coplanar	hysteresis	strain energy
creep	load	stress
damping	mechanical fatigue	stress relaxation
dashpot	modulus of elasticity	tension
deform	plastic range	three-point principle
ductile	plasticity	torsional load

Suggested Reading List

Adams MA. Biomechanics of back pain. *Acupunct Med.* 2004;22:178-188.

Adams MA, Green TP, Dolan P. The strength in anterior bending of lumbar intervertebral discs. *Spine (Phila Pa 1976).* 1994;19:2197-2203.

Adams MA, Hutton WC. The mechanical function of the lumbar apophyseal joints. *Spine (Phila Pa 1976).* 1983;8:327-330.

Arampatzis A, Stafilidis S, DeMonte G, Karamanidis K, Morey-Klapsing G, Bruggemann GP. Strain and elongation of the human gastrocnemius tendon and aponeurosis during maximal plantarflexion effort. *J Biomech.* 2005;38:833-841.

Beaupre GS, Stevens SS, Carter DR. Mechanobiology in the development, maintenance, and degeneration of articular cartilage. *J Rehabil Res Dev.* 2000;37:145-151.

Benhardt H, Cosgriff-Hernandez E. The role of mechanical loading in ligament tissue engineering. *Tissue Eng Part B Rev.* 2009.

Benjamin M, Ralphs JR. Tendons and ligaments—an overview. *Histol Histopathol.* 1997;12:1135-1144.

Benjamin M, Toumi H, Ralphs JR, Bydder G, Best TM, Milz S. Where tendons and ligaments meet bone: attachment sites ('entheses') in relation to exercise and/or mechanical load. *J Anat.* 2006;208:471-490.

Butler DL, Goldstein SA, Guldberg RE, et al. The impact of biomechanics in tissue engineering and regenerative medicine. *Tissue Eng Part B Rev.* 2009;15(4):477-484.

Carter DR, Beaupre GS. *Skeletal Function and Form: Mechanobiology of Skeletal Development, Aging, and Regeneration.* New York, NY: Cambridge University Press; 2001.

Carter DR, Beaupre GS, Wong M, Smith RL, Andriacchi TP, Schurman DJ. The mechanobiology of articular cartilage development and degeneration. *Clin Orthop Relat Res.* 2004:S69-S77.

Chaffin DB, Andersson GBJ, Martin BJ. *Occupational Biomechanics.* 4th ed. Hoboken, NJ: John Wiley & Sons, Inc; 2006.

Daly RM. The effect of exercise on bone mass and structural geometry during growth. *Med Sport Sci.* 2007;51:33-49.

Dibb AT, Nightingale RW, Luck JF, Chancey VC, Fronheiser LE, Myers BS. Tension and combined tension-extension structural response and tolerance properties of the human male ligamentous cervical spine. *J Biomech Eng.* 2009;131(8):081008.

Duggal N, Pickett GE, Mitsis DK, Keller JL. Early clinical and biomechanical results following cervical arthroplasty. *Neurosurg Focus*. 2004;17:E9.

Ebara S, Iatridis JC, Setton LA, Foster RJ, Mow VC, Weidenbaum M. Tensile properties of nondegenerate human lumbar anulus fibrosus. *Spine (Phila Pa 1976)*. 1996;21:452-461.

Enderle J, Blanchard S, Bronzino J. *Introduction to Biomedical Engineering*. 2nd ed. Burlington, MA: Elsevier Academic Press Series; 2005.

Frelinghuysen P, Huang RC, Girardi FP, Cammisa FP Jr. Lumbar total disc replacement part I: rationale, biomechanics, and implant types. *Orthop Clin North Am*. 2005;36:293-299.

Frost HM. Bone's mechanostat: a 2003 update. *Anat Rec A Discov Mol Cell Evol Biol*. 2003;275:1081-1101.

Frost HM. Muscle, bone, and the Utah paradigm: a 1999 overview. *Med Sci Sports Exerc*. 2000;32:911-917.

Frost HM. On the strength-safety factor (SSF) for load-bearing skeletal organs. *J Musculoskelet Neuronal Interact*. 2003;3:136-140.

Frost HM. The Utah paradigm of skeletal physiology: an overview of its insights for bone, cartilage and collagenous tissue organs. *J Bone Miner Metab*. 2000;18:305-316.

Fung YC. *Biomechanics: Mechanical Properties of Living Tissues*. 2nd ed. New York, NY: Georg Thieme Verlag; 1997.

Galbusera F, Bellini CM, Zweig T, et al. Design concepts in lumbar total disc arthroplasty. *Eur Spine J*. 2008;17:1635-1650.

Gupte CM, Smith A, Jamieson N, Bull AM, Thomas RD, Amis AA. Meniscofemoral ligaments—structural and material properties. *J Biomech*. 2002;35:1623-1629.

Hadjipavlou AG, Tzermiadianos MN, Bogduk N, Zindrick MR. The pathophysiology of disc degeneration: a critical review. *J Bone Joint Surg Br*. 2008;90:1261-1270.

Halder A, Zobitz ME, Schultz E, An KN. Structural properties of the subscapularis tendon. *J Orthop Res*. 2000;18:829-834.

Henderson JH, Carter DR. Mechanical induction in limb morphogenesis: the role of growth-generated strains and pressures. *Bone*. 2002;31:645-653.

Henderson JH, de la Fuente L, Romero D, et al. Rapid growth of cartilage rudiments may generate perichondrial structures by mechanical induction. *Biomech Model Mechanobiol*. 2007;6:127-137.

Heuer F, Schmidt H, Wilke HJ. The relation between intervertebral disc bulging and annular fiber associated strains for simple and complex loading. *J Biomech*. 2008;41:1086-1094.

Hill PA. Bone remodelling. *Br J Orthod*. 1998;25:101-107.

Huang RC, Wright TM, Panjabi MM, Lipman JD. Biomechanics of nonfusion implants. *Orthop Clin North Am*. 2005;36:271-280.

Hukins DW, Kirby MC, Sikoryn TA, Aspden RM, Cox AJ. Comparison of structure, mechanical properties, and functions of lumbar spinal ligaments. *Spine (Phila Pa 1976)*. 1990;15:787-795.

Iatridis JC, Kumar S, Foster RJ, Weidenbaum M, Mow VC. Shear mechanical properties of human lumbar annulus fibrosus. *J Orthop Res*. 1999;17:732-737.

Iatridis JC, Setton LA, Weidenbaum M, Mow VC. The viscoelastic behavior of the non-degenerate human lumbar nucleus pulposus in shear. *J Biomech*. 1997;30:1005-1013.

Itoi E, Berglund LJ, Grabowski JJ, et al. Tensile properties of the supraspinatus tendon. *J Orthop Res*. 1995;13:578-584.

James R, Kesturu G, Balian G, Chhabra AB. Tendon: biology, biomechanics, repair, growth factors, and evolving treatment options. *J Hand Surg Am*. 2008;33:102-112.

Janz KF, Gilmore JM, Levy SM, Letuchy EM, Burns TL, Beck TJ. Physical activity and femoral neck bone strength during childhood: the Iowa Bone Development Study. *Bone*. 2007;41:216-222.

Jonkers I, Sauwen N, Lenaerts G, Mulier M, Van der Perre G, Jaecques S. Relation between subject-specific hip joint loading, stress distribution in the proximal femur and bone mineral density changes after total hip replacement. *J Biomech*. 2008;41:3405-3413.

Jung HJ, Fisher MB, Woo SL. Role of biomechanics in the understanding of normal, injured, and healing ligaments and tendons. *Sports Med Arthrosc Rehabil Ther Technol*. 2009;1:9.

Karinkanta S, Heinonen A, Sievanen H, Uusi-Rasi K, Fogelholm M, Kannus P. Maintenance of exercise-induced benefits in physical functioning and bone among elderly women. *Osteoporos Int.* 2009;20:665-674.

Kjaer M. Role of extracellular matrix in adaptation of tendon and skeletal muscle to mechanical loading. *Physiol Rev.* 2004;84:649-698.

Kjaer M, Magnusson P, Krogsgaard M, et al. Extracellular matrix adaptation of tendon and skeletal muscle to exercise. *J Anat.* 2006;208:445-450.

Kontulainen SA, Hughes JM, Macdonald HM, Johnston JD. The biomechanical basis of bone strength development during growth. *Med Sport Sci.* 2007;51:13-32.

Koob TJ. Biomimetic approaches to tendon repair. *Comp Biochem Physiol A Mol Integr Physiol.* 2002;133:1171-1192.

Kristiansen LP. Reconstructive surgery of the human tibia by use of external ring fixator and the Ilizarov method. *Acta Orthop Suppl.* 2009;80:1-43.

Lieber RL, Murray WM, Clark DL, Hentz VR, Friden J. Biomechanical properties of the brachioradialis muscle: Implications for surgical tendon transfer. *J Hand Surg Am.* 2005;30:273-282.

Maganaris CN. Tensile properties of in vivo human tendinous tissue. *J Biomech.* 2002;35:1019-1027.

Maganaris CN, Narici MV, Maffulli N. Biomechanics of the Achilles tendon. *Disabil Rehabil.* 2008;30:1542-1547.

Maganaris CN, Paul JP. Hysteresis measurements in intact human tendon. *J Biomech.* 2000;33:1723-1727.

Maganaris CN, Reeves ND, Rittweger J, et al. Adaptive response of human tendon to paralysis. *Muscle Nerve.* 2006;33:85-92.

Martin RB, Burr DB, Sharkey NA. *Skeletal Tissue Mechanics.* New York, NY: Springer-Verlag; 1998.

McGough RL, Debski RE, Taskiran E, Fu FH, Woo SL. Mechanical properties of the long head of the biceps tendon. *Knee Surg Sports Traumatol Arthrosc.* 1996;3:226-229.

Miller ME. The bone disease of preterm birth: a biomechanical perspective. *Pediatr Res.* 2003;53:10-15.

Miller ME. Hypothesis: fetal movement influences fetal and infant bone strength. *Med Hypotheses.* 2005;65:880-886.

Muramatsu T, Muraoka T, Takeshita D, Kawakami Y, Hirano Y, Fukunaga T. Mechanical properties of tendon and aponeurosis of human gastrocnemius muscle in vivo. *J Appl Physiol.* 2001;90:1671-1678.

Musahl V, Lehner A, Watanabe Y, Fu FH. Biology and biomechanics. *Curr Opin Rheumatol.* 2002;14:127-133.

Myklebust JB, Pintar F, Yoganandan N, et al. Tensile strength of spinal ligaments. *Spine (Phila Pa 1976).* 1988;13:526-531.

Narici MV, Maffulli N, Maganaris CN. Ageing of human muscles and tendons. *Disabil Rehabil.* 2008;30:1548-1554.

Narici MV, Maganaris CN. Adaptability of elderly human muscles and tendons to increased loading. *J Anat.* 2006;208:433-443.

Oostenbroek HJ, Brand R, van Roermund PM. Lower limb deformity due to failed trauma treatment corrected with the Ilizarov technique. *Acta Orthop.* 2009:80(4):435-439.

Ouyang J, Zhu Q, Zhao W, Xu Y, Chen W, Zhong S. Biomechanical assessment of the pediatric cervical spine under bending and tensile loading. *Spine (Phila Pa 1976).* 2005;30:E716-E723.

Palomares KT, Gleason RE, Mason ZD, et al. Mechanical stimulation alters tissue differentiation and molecular expression during bone healing. *J Orthop Res.* 2009;27:1123-1132.

Pearson OM, Lieberman DE. The aging of Wolff's "law": ontogeny and responses to mechanical loading in cortical bone. *Am J Phys Anthropol.* 2004;Suppl 39:63-99.

Reeves ND. Adaptation of the tendon to mechanical usage. *J Musculoskelet Neuronal Interact.* 2006;6:174-180.

Reich A, Sharir A, Zelzer E, Hacker L, Monsonego-Ornan E, Shahar R. The effect of weight loading and subsequent release from loading on the postnatal skeleton. *Bone.* 2008;43:766-774.

Rittweger J. Ten years muscle-bone hypothesis: what have we learned so far?—almost a festschrift—. *J Musculoskelet Neuronal Interact.* 2008;8:174-178.

Robling AG, Castillo AB, Turner CH. Biomechanical and molecular regulation of bone remodeling. *Annu Rev Biomed Eng.* 2006;8:455-498.

Sasso RC, Best NM. Cervical kinematics after fusion and bryan disc arthroplasty. *J Spinal Disord Tech.* 2008;21:19-22.

Seeman E. The structural and biomechanical basis of the gain and loss of bone strength in women and men. *Endocrinol Metab Clin North Am.* 2003;32:25-38.

Seeman E. Structural basis of growth-related gain and age-related loss of bone strength. *Rheumatology (Oxford).* 2008;47 Suppl 4:iv2-8.

Setton LA, Chen J. Cell mechanics and mechanobiology in the intervertebral disc. *Spine (Phila Pa 1976).* 2004;29:2710-2723.

Setton LA, Chen J. Mechanobiology of the intervertebral disc and relevance to disc degeneration. *J Bone Joint Surg Am.* 2006;88 Suppl 2:52-57.

Shefelbine SJ, Carter DR. Mechanobiological predictions of femoral anteversion in cerebral palsy. *Ann Biomed Eng.* 2004;32:297-305.

Shefelbine SJ, Carter DR. Mechanobiological predictions of growth front morphology in developmental hip dysplasia. *J Orthop Res.* 2004;22:346-352.

Smith EL, Gilligan C. Dose-response relationship between physical loading and mechanical competence of bone. *Bone.* 1996;18:455-505.

Solomonow M. Ligaments: a source of musculoskeletal disorders. *J Bodyw Mov Ther.* 2009;13:136-154.

Solomonow M. Ligaments: a source of work-related musculoskeletal disorders. *J Electromyogr Kinesiol.* 2004;14:49-60.

Stokes IA. Mechanical effects on skeletal growth. *J Musculoskelet Neuronal Interact.* 2002;2:277-280.

Stokes IA, Clark KC, Farnum CE, Aronsson DD. Alterations in the growth plate associated with growth modulation by sustained compression or distraction. *Bone.* 2007;41:197-205.

Taylor RE, Zheng C, Jackson RP, et al. The phenomenon of twisted growth: humeral torsion in dominant arms of high performance tennis players. *Comput Methods Biomech Biomed Engin.* 2009;12:83-93.

Thomopoulos S, Williams GR, Gimbel JA, Favata M, Soslowsky LJ. Variation of biomechanical, structural, and compositional properties along the tendon to bone insertion site. *J Orthop Res.* 2003;21:413-419.

Turner CH. Bone strength: current concepts. *Ann N Y Acad Sci.* 2006;1068:429-446.

Turner CH. Three rules for bone adaptation to mechanical stimuli. *Bone.* 1998;23:399-407.

Turner CH, Robling AG. Mechanisms by which exercise improves bone strength. *J Bone Miner Metab.* 2005;23 Suppl:16-22.

Turner CH, Warden SJ, Bellido T, et al. Mechanobiology of the skeleton. *Sci Signal.* 2009;2:pt3.

Villemure I, Stokes IA. Growth plate mechanics and mechanobiology. A survey of present understanding. *J Biomech.* 2009;42:1793-1803.

Voudouris JC, Kuftinec MM. Improved clinical use of Twin-block and Herbst as a result of radiating viscoelastic tissue forces on the condyle and fossa in treatment and long-term retention: growth relativity. *Am J Orthod Dentofacial Orthop.* 2000;117:247-266.

Wang JH. Mechanobiology of tendon. *J Biomech.* 2006;39:1563-1582.

Ward KA, Caulton JM, Adams JE, Mughal MZ. Perspective: cerebral palsy as a model of bone development in the absence of postnatal mechanical factors. *J Musculoskelet Neuronal Interact.* 2006;6:154-159.

Ward SR, Tomiya A, Regev GJ, et al. Passive mechanical properties of the lumbar multifidus muscle support its role as a stabilizer. *J Biomech.* 2009;42:1384-1389.

Wendlova J. Bone quality. Elasticity and strength. *Bratisl Lek Listy.* 2008;109:383-386.

Wnek GE, Bowlin GL. *Encyclopedia of Biomaterials and Biomedical Engineering.* New York, NY: Marcel Dekker, Inc.; 2004.

Westh E, Kongsgaard M, Bojsen-Moller J, et al. Effect of habitual exercise on the structural and mechanical properties of human tendon, in vivo, in men and women. *Scand J Med Sci Sports.* 2008;18:23-30.

Wilke HJ, Rohlmann A, Neller S, et al. Is it possible to simulate physiologic loading conditions by applying pure moments? A comparison of in vivo and in vitro load components in an internal fixator. *Spine (Phila Pa 1976).* 2001;26:636-642.

Woo SL, Abramowitch SD, Kilger R, Liang R. Biomechanics of knee ligaments: injury, healing, and repair. *J Biomech.* 2006;39:1-20.

Woo SL, Fisher MB, Feola AJ. Contribution of biomechanics to management of ligament and tendon injuries. *Mol Cell Biomech.* 2008;5:49-68.

Wren TA, Beaupre GS, Carter DR. Tendon and ligament adaptation to exercise, immobilization, and remobilization. *J Rehabil Res Dev.* 2000;37:217-224.

Wren TA, Lindsey DP, Beaupre GS, Carter DR. Effects of creep and cyclic loading on the mechanical properties and failure of human Achilles tendons. *Ann Biomed Eng.* 2003;31:710-717.

Yamamoto S, Hagiwara A, Mizobe T, Yokoyama O, Yasui T. Development of an ankle-foot orthosis with an oil damper. *Prosthet Orthot Int.* 2005;29:209-219.

Yokoyama O, Sashika H, Hagiwara A, Yamamoto S, Yasui T. Kinematic effects on gait of a newly designed ankle-foot orthosis with oil damper resistance: a case series of 2 patients with hemiplegia. *Arch Phys Med Rehabil.* 2005;86:162-166.

Zhang P, Hamamura K, Yokota H. A brief review of bone adaptation to unloading. *Genomics Proteomics Bioinformatics.* 2008;6:4-7.

chapter 3

Composition and Resolution of Forces

Objectives

1. Define and compare composition and resolution.
2. Define collinear, concurrent, concentric, and coplanar.
3. Draw the resultants and components of selected forces.
4. Determine the resultant of 2 or more forces.
5. Calculate the components of a given force.
6. Provide and discuss examples of composition and resolution of forces in the body, in clinical use, and in everyday activities.

Introduction

To understand the effects of forces on an object, we must take into account all of the forces that are acting upon it. The situation may consist of analyzing a single force system or a combination of force systems. Once we know the types and characteristics of the forces involved, we can determine how these forces affect and react to the human body.

Innumerable examples of composition and resolution exist in everyday life. As each muscle contracts, it can be separated into force components that act perpendicular and parallel to the limb. As the quadriceps muscles pull on the patella, the patella can be moved laterally and posteriorly. If 2 or more muscles are acting across a joint, their combined effect can be determined. The tension, shearing, and compression effects in joints result from separating the force in the joint into its components. The initial contact, stance, and push off of the foot can be separated into forces perpendicular and parallel to the supporting surface. Knowledge of the direction and magnitude of force components or of the result of combined forces provides information useful in determining the cause and extent of injury. Treatment of hand injuries and deformities, treatments for facial growth modification, manual forces acting for mobilization, traction treatments, and force components of exercise treatments must all use information related to composition and resolution.

Thus, forces can be combined to provide a single resulting force, or one force can be separated into its perpendicular components. The process of combining forces is called the composition of forces, while the process of separating 1 force into 2 components is called resolution of forces.

LeVeau BF.
Biomechanics of Human Motion: Basics and Beyond for the Health Professions (pp 55-70).
© 2011 SLACK Incorporated

Composition

Often, a set of several forces acts simultaneously on an object. These forces arriving from different directions may be replaced by a single force, which will have the same effect as that of the set of forces. This single force that results is called the resultant of the forces. The process of composition of forces can be shown either graphically or mathematically.

Graphic Method (Triangular)

Because forces are vectors (quantities having both magnitude and direction), the graphic method uses precise measurements of magnitude and direction of the involved forces to obtain the resulting force (Figure 3-1). The forces are represented by arrows; the length of the arrow indicates the magnitude of the force, the shaft shows its line of action, and the arrowhead illustrates its direction. The arrows are drawn end to end. The first arrow begins at a point representing the point of application. The tail of each successive arrow is placed at the head of the preceding arrow. When all of the arrows are drawn, the resultant is determined by an arrow with its tail at the point of application and its head at the tip of the last connected arrow. If the individual arrows are drawn precisely, the magnitude, line of application, and direction of the resultant are displayed.

Graphic Method (Parallelogram)

The parallelogram method (Figure 3-2) takes 2 forces at a time (A and B). The 2 force vectors are both drawn with the tails of the arrows at the same point of origin. A dotted line representing force B is then drawn with its tail at the head of force A. A dotted line representing force A is drawn with its tail at the head of force B. If the vectors have been drawn correctly to scale for magnitude and direction, the resulting figure should be a parallelogram. The diagonal from the point of origin to where the heads of the dotted lines meet represents the resultant of the 2 forces. The length of the diagonal line is the magnitude of the force; the angle between the diagonal line and one of the given forces provides the line of application; and an arrowhead on the diagonal line where the 2 heads of the dotted lines meet gives the direction.

Mathematical Method

The resultant can also be determined by use of algebra and trigonometry. However, a diagram of the forces is needed to help understand the solution of the problem. If only 2 forces are acting on the object, the Cosine Law can be used to calculate the magnitude of the resultant force (Figure 3-3). To find the resultant of several forces, the equation may be used taking 2 forces at a time.

$$R = \sqrt{A^2 + B^2 - 2AB\cos\Phi}$$

Note that the angle Φ is the angle between the 2 forces as they are placed tail to head and not the angle between the 2 forces at the point of origin.

Once the 3 sides and one angle are known from the Cosine Law, the remaining 2 angles can be determined by using the Cosine Law for each unknown angle. Be sure to use the appropriate sides with the included angle. Also, the Sine Law may be used (Figure 3-4).

$$\frac{A}{\sin\alpha} = \frac{B}{\sin\beta} = \frac{R}{\sin\Phi}$$

If the angle between the 2 forces is 90 degrees, then the equation becomes what is known as the Pythagorean Theorem, or

$$R = \sqrt{A^2 + B^2}$$

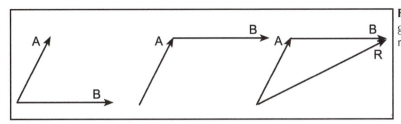

Figure 3-1. Graphic (triangular) method to obtain the resulting force.

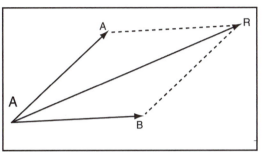

Figure 3-2. Graphic (parallelogram) method to obtain the resulting force.

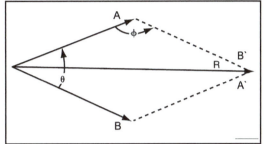

Figure 3-3. Cosine law to calculate the magnitude of the resultant force.

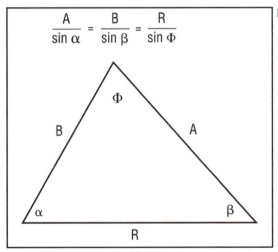

Figure 3-4. Law of Sines: $\frac{A}{\sin\alpha} = \frac{B}{\sin\beta} = \frac{C}{\sin\phi}$.

In this situation, the angle for the line of application of the resultant can be calculated using the inverse tangent.

$$\Phi = \tan^{-1}\left(\frac{B}{A}\right)$$

LINEAR FORCE SYSTEM

A system of forces can be considered a linear force system when all of the forces lie on the same line (collinear) and in the same plane (coplanar).

A vertical weight rack (Figure 3-5) is holding 2 dumbbells, one weighing 10 lb and the other 5 lb. What is their resultant weight? We know that for each weight the point of application is on the rack one above the other, the line of application is vertical, the direction is downward, and the magnitudes have been given. To solve this problem graphically, we can draw a vector for the 5-lb weight followed by a vector for the 10-lb weight with a scale of 0.25 in for each lb. The resultant of the 2 forces would be 3.75 in or 15 lb.

Figure 3-5. A vertical weight rack holding weights represents a linear force system.

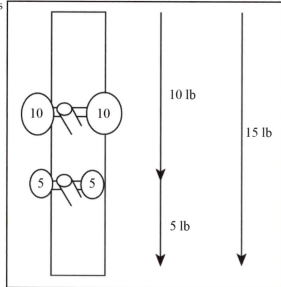

Solving this problem mathematically appears to be very simple by adding the magnitudes of 10 lb and 5 lb to obtain 15 lb. We could use the Cosine Law to determine the resultant as follows. Note in the figure that the angle between the 2 forces is 180 degrees. Therefore, the cos 180 degrees is equal to -1.

$$R^2 = A^2 + B^2 - 2ABcos\Phi$$

$$R^2 = (10 \text{ lb})^2 + (5 \text{ lb})^2 - (2)(10 \text{ lb})(5 \text{ lb})(\cos 180 \text{ degrees})$$

$$R^2 = 100 \text{ lb} + 25 \text{ lb} + 100 \text{ lb}$$

$$R^2 = 225 \text{ lb}$$

$$R = 15 \text{ lb}$$

CONCURRENT FORCE SYSTEM

A system of forces can be considered a concurrent force system when all of the forces concur or meet at the same point (concurrent) and lie in the same plane (coplanar), but do not act along the same line.

Suppose we would like to determine the resultant of a traction system pulling on the leg (Figure 3-6). Because the 20-lb weight transmits 20 lb of tension throughout the cord, the 2 forces of the traction system acting on the leg are equal to 20 lb each. The system is set up so that the angle between the 2 forces is 60 degrees.

The graphic approach is shown in Figure 3-6E. The figure may be drawn as a triangle or a parallelogram. Careful attention to drawing the angles accurately and the line lengths to scale should provide a resultant of approximately 34.6 lb.

The results using the mathematical method should confirm the answer of the graphic method. We may use the Cosine Law to determine the resultant as follows. Note in Figure 3-7 that the angle between the 2 forces for using the Cosine Law is 120 degrees, not 60 degrees. The cos 120 degrees is equal to -0.5.

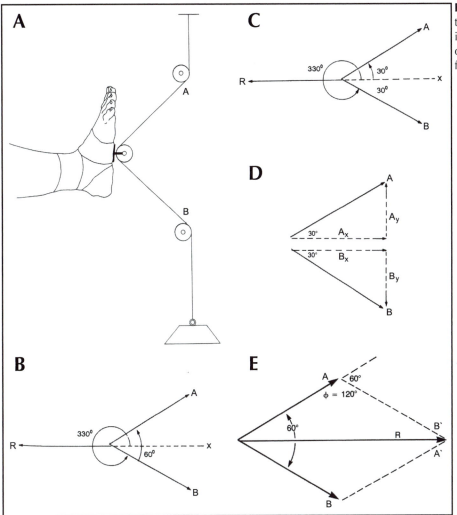

Figure 3-6. A traction system is an example of a concurrent force system.

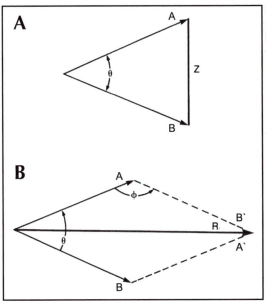

Figure 3-7. Use of cosine law for determination of resultant forces A and B. (A) Using θ as the angle between A and B does not provide the proper resultant value. (B) Shows the appropriate resultant vector.

$$R^2 = A^2 + B^2 - 2AB\cos\Phi$$

$$R^2 = (20 \text{ lb})^2 + (20 \text{ lb})^2 - (2)(20 \text{ lb})(20 \text{ lb})(\cos 120 \text{ degrees})$$

$$R^2 = 400 \text{ lb} + 400 \text{ lb} + 400 \text{ lb}$$

$$R^2 = 1200 \text{ lb}$$

$$R = 34.46 \text{ lb}$$

Because the 2 acting forces are equal in this situation, the resultant will bisect them. Therefore, the resultant is 30 degrees from each acting force. The Sine Law confirms the value of the angle as shown:

$$\frac{A}{\sin\alpha} = \frac{B}{\sin\beta} = \frac{R}{\sin\Phi}$$

$$\frac{20 \text{ lb}}{\sin\alpha} = \frac{34.64 \text{ lb}}{\sin 120 \text{ degrees}}$$

$$\frac{(20 \text{ lb} \times \sin 120 \text{ degrees})}{34.64 \text{ lb}} = \sin\alpha$$

$$\frac{(20 \text{ lb} \times 0.866)}{34.64 \text{ lb}} = \sin\alpha$$

$$0.5 = \sin\alpha$$

$$\alpha = 30 \text{ degrees}$$

The equation would also show that the angle α would equal 30 degrees.

In a special situation in which the 2 forces act perpendicular to each other, the Pythagorean Theorem may be used. Suppose a 50-lb force is acting vertically and a 100-lb force is acting horizontally (Figure 3-8), we can find the resultant in the following manner:

$$R = \sqrt{A^2 + B^2}$$

$$R = \sqrt{(50 \text{ lb})^2 + (100)^2}$$

$$R = \sqrt{2500 + 10,000}$$

$$R = \sqrt{12,500}$$

$$R = 111.8 \text{ lb}$$

The angle for the line of application is found as follows.

The resulting force has a magnitude of 111.8 lb at 26.56 degrees with the horizontal.

$$\tan\Theta = \frac{50 \text{ lb}}{100 \text{ lb}}$$

$$\tan\Theta = 0.5$$

$$\Theta = 26.56 \text{ degrees}$$

Note that the linear and concurrent systems were solved the same way. In fact, the linear system can be considered a special case of the concurrent system in which the forces act along the same line. When we have 2 or more forces acting on a point, the magnitude of the result can range between zero and the sum of the forces. For example, if 2 equal forces act together in the same direction, the maximum resultant magnitude will be the sum of the magnitudes of the 2 forces. However, if the 2 equal forces act in opposite directions, the resultant will be zero. As the angle between 2 forces decreases from 180 degrees to 0 degrees, their resultant increases. Note that this angle is not the same angle as used in the Cosine Law calculations, but is the angle taken between the lines of application originating from their point of concurrence (Figure 3-9).

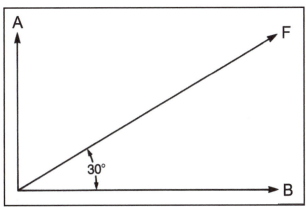

Figure 3-8. Composition when the 2 forces are perpendicular to each other.

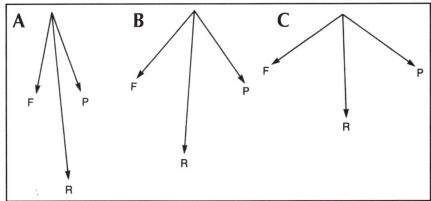

Figure 3-9. Decrease in the magnitude of the resultant as the angle between the force vectors increases. At 0 degrees, the resultant is greatest, and at 180 degrees, the resultant is the least.

Several examples of composition exist within the human body. Whenever 2 or more muscles act in a synergistic manner, composition must be considered. At the knee joint, the 4 quadriceps muscles produce one resulting force (Figure 3-10). This resulting force in the frontal plane combined with the opposing patellar tendon force on the patella may tend to laterally sublux the patella (Figure 3-11). The resulting force in the sagittal plane combined with the opposing patellar tendon force on the patella put a compressive force on the femoral condyles (Figure 3-12). At the hip, 3 heads of the gluteus medius, the gluteus minimus, and the tensor fascia lata combine to create one resulting force (Figure 3-13). Similarly, the 2 heads of the gastrocnemius develop a single resultant (Figure 3-14). The fibers of a bipennate muscle combine to produce a resulting muscle force (Figure 3-15).

Resolution

The process of resolution separates a force into its 2 perpendicular components (Figure 3-16). This process can also be done graphically or mathematically. The selection of the line of application for the components is very important in the determination of the effects of the acting force. An important example is the resolution of muscle force as it acts on the body (Figure 3-17). The lines of application should be perpendicular and parallel to the bone on which the muscle is acting. The perpendicular component (R, or y) is the force component that tends to cause the bone to rotate around the adjacent joint. The parallel or tangent component (NR, or x) determines the magnitude of force directed toward or away from the adjacent joint and is a non-rotatory force.

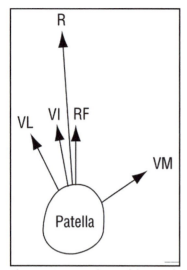

Figure 3-10. Resultant of the quadriceps muscle.

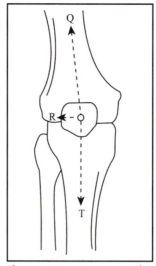

Figure 3-11. Forces on the patella in the frontal plane.

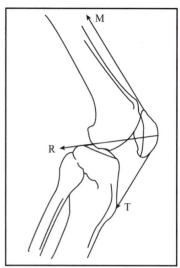

Figure 3-12. Forces on the patella in the sagittal plane.

Figure 3-13. (A) Hip abductor muscles. (Adapted from Gottschalk F, Kourosh S, LeVeau B. The functional anatomy of tensor fasciae latae and gluteus medius and minimus. *J Anat.* 1989;166:179-189.) (B) Force vectors and resultant of the hip abductor muscles. (Adapted from Inman VT. Functional aspects of the abductor muscles of the hip. *J Bone Joint Surg.* 1947;29:607-619.)

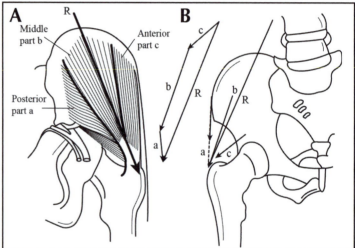

Figure 3-14. Medial (M) and lateral (L) heads of the gastrocnemius muscle together pull upward on the tendon of Achilles.

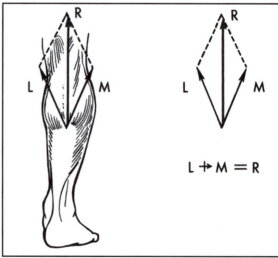

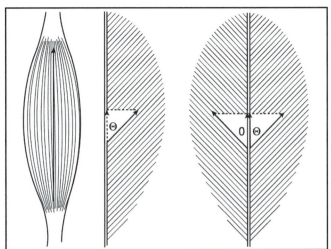

Figure 3-15. Resultant muscle force from muscle fiber force vectors.

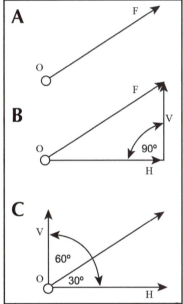

Figure 3-16. Determination of the rectangular force components of the force F acting at a 30-degree angle. (A) Force F is acting at point O. (B) Perpendicular components H and V are drawn end to end from O to the tip of F. (C) Force component V is moved to the point of application.

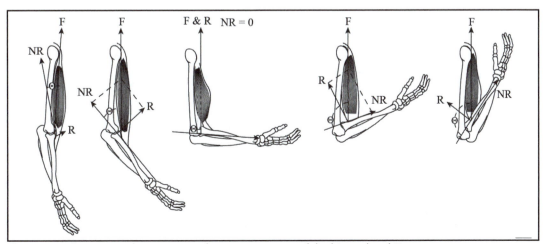

Figure 3-17. Rotatory and non-rotatory force components of the biceps brachii.

GRAPHIC METHOD

In the graphic method, the components should be drawn perpendicular to each other along the appropriate lines of application directed from the point of application to obtain a triangle or a rectangle (see Figure 3-16). Once this graphic display is made, one of the component force arrows should be constructed so that its arrowhead is placed at the head of the original force and its tail at the head of the other component to produce a right triangle in which the lengths of the sides represent the magnitude of force components. The hypotenuse represents the magnitude, line of application, and direction of the original force.

MATHEMATICAL METHOD

The mathematical determination of these force components uses the right triangle approach. The relationship of the force vectors is determined by using the trigonometric functions of sine, cosine, and tangent:

- sine = opposite side/hypotenuse
- cosine = adjacent side/hypotenuse
- tangent = opposite side/adjacent side

Example: Suppose we would like to find the vertical (y component) and horizontal (x component) force components of a 100-lb force acting at a 30 degree angle (see Figure 3-16A). Graphically, the solution can be performed by drawing a triangle or rectangle using the given force as the diagonal of the rectangle and measuring all lines to scale (see Figures 3-16B and 3-16C). The mathematical solution must use trigonometric functions as follows:

$$\frac{F_x}{F} = \cos\Theta$$

$$F_x = F \cos 30 \text{ degrees}$$

$$F_x = 100 \text{ lb} \times 0.866$$

$$F_x = 86.6 \text{ lb}$$

$$\frac{F_y}{F} = \sin\alpha$$

$$F_y = F \sin 30 \text{ degrees}$$

$$F_y = 100 \text{ lb} \times 0.5$$

$$F_y = 50 \text{ lb}$$

The horizontal force component is 86.6 lb, and the vertical force component is 50 lb. In this situation, the horizontal component is 86.6% of the acting force, and the vertical component is 50% of the acting force. Note that the percentages of the total magnitude are greater than 100% because the forces are vectors and not scalar.

Every force can be resolved into perpendicular components. Muscles pulling on a bone (Figure 3-18) have a component that causes rotation (rotatory component perpendicular to the bone) and a component that causes stress on the joint (non-rotatory component parallel to the bone). Forces such as foot contact (Figure 3-19), a tilt table (Figure 3-20), exercise devices (Figure 3-21), traction (Figure 3-22), and gravity on a body part (Figures 3-23 and 3-24) all can be separated into perpendicular components.

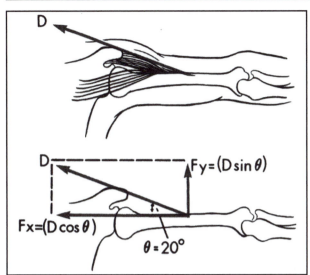

Figure 3-18. Resolution of deltoid muscle force into rotatory (F_y) and non-rotatory (F_x) components.

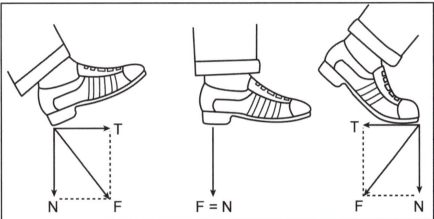

Figure 3-19. Perpendicular force components of foot contact.

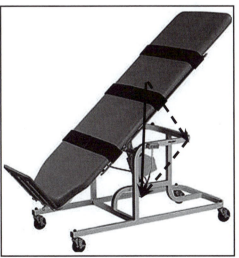

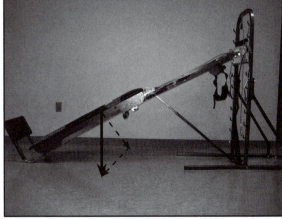

Figure 3-21. Perpendicular force components of Total Gym.

Figure 3-20. Perpendicular force components of a tilt table. Reprinted with permission from Patterson Medical/Sammons Preston, Bolingbrook, IL.

Figure 3-22. Perpendicular force components of cervical traction.

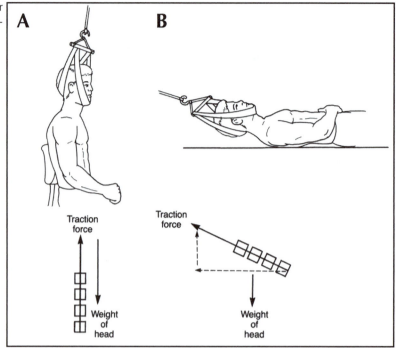

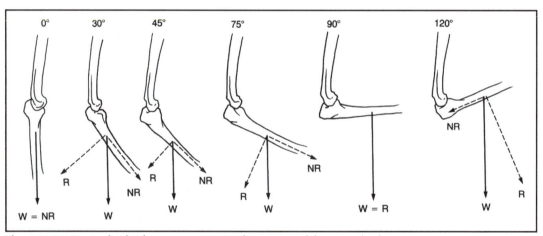

Figure 3-23. Perpendicular force components of gravitational force on the forearm.

Figure 3-24. Change in the compression and shearing force components with the change in the sacral angle.

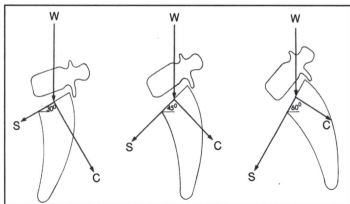

Activities

1. Define the following terms.

collinear	coplanar	resultant
composition	linear force system	sine
concentric	parallel component	Sine law
concurrent force system	perpendicular component	tangent
cosine	resolution	tangential component
Cosine law		

2. Provide and discuss examples of composition and resolution of forces in the body, in clinical use, and in everyday activities.

3. Draw the force components of the following situations:

   a. Vertical (normal) and horizontal (tangential) components by the foot at push off. Explain the differences that occur with change in speed.

   b. Perpendicular components of an individual's center of mass on a tilt table. (Do for angles of 0 degrees, 30 degrees, 45 degrees, and 60 degrees.)

   c. The rotatory and non-rotatory components of an elastic band used for knee extension. (Do for angles of 90 degrees, 60 degrees, 45 degrees, 30 degrees, and 0 degrees.)

4. Which requires stronger ropes to support a 150-lb person, a swing or a hammock?

5. What is the force on the cord supporting a 40-lb tennis net if the cord forms an 85 degree angle with the supporting pole? Why is a cable used for this?

6. A 150-lb athlete sitting on an exercise table with the knee relaxed at 90 degrees has a 30-lb cuff on his ankle. If his leg and foot weigh 9 lb, what is the load on the soft tissues of the knee? Is the load producing tension, compression, or shearing in the collateral ligaments?

7. Find the horizontal and vertical components of a 10-lb force acting at a 30 degree angle with the horizontal.

8. What percentage of the muscle force effectively produces rotatory motion if the muscle inserts at an angle of 30 degrees; 45 degrees; 60 degrees? What percentage of the force at each angle is non-rotatory?

9. How does the resultant change as the angle between 2 concurrent forces decreases? Increases? What angle provides the maximum resultant? Minimum resultant?

10. A girl wishes to canoe across a river having a velocity of 8 miles per hour. If she starts straight across the river at 5 miles per hour, what is the angle that she travels with the bank of the river? If the river is 400-ft wide, what distance downstream will she travel before reaching the opposite bank?

11. Describe the patellofemoral joint force as an individual moves from an upright stance to a squat position. Relate this to going up and down stairs.

12. Describe how the component forces of the body weight above the sacrum change as the sacral angle changes.

13. Draw and calculate the gravitational force components of a 10-lb upper limb with shoulder abduction of 0 degrees; 30 degrees; 45 degrees; 60 degrees; 90 degrees; 120 degrees.

14. Draw and calculate the muscle force components of the brachialis exerting 50 lb of force flexing the elbow at 0 degrees; 30 degrees; 45 degrees; 60 degrees; 90 degrees; 120 degrees.

15. Draw and calculate the muscle force components of the hamstring muscles exerting 100 lb of force flexing the elbow at 0 degrees; 30 degrees; 45 degrees; 60 degrees; 90 degrees.

16. The 4 quadriceps muscles pull on the patella simultaneously. They apply forces as follows (the angles are measured in the frontal plane):

    Vastus lateralis: 170 lb at angle of 30 degrees to the left of vertical

    Rectus femoris: 55 lb at angle of 16 degrees to the left of vertical

    Vastus intermedius: 155 lb at angle of 15 degrees to the left of vertical

    Vastus medialis: 120 lb at angle of 35 degrees to the right of vertical

    a. What is their resultant force?

    b. If the patellar tendon attaches at 0 degrees with vertical, what is the resultant force on the patella?

    c. What would happen if the tibial tuberosity were surgically moved medially so that the patellar tendon attaches at 12 degrees with vertical?

    d. Instead of the surgical intervention, what would happen if the vastus medialis was strengthened or trained to contract with 180 lb of force?

ANSWERS

4. Hammock

5. 229 lb

6. 39 lb, tension

7. Horizontal = 8.66 lb; vertical = 5 lb

8. R: 50%, 70.7%, 86.7% NR: 86.7%. 70.7%, 50%

9. It increases; 0 degrees; 180 degrees

10. 32 degrees, 640 ft

13.

Angle	R	NR
0 degrees	0 lb	10 lb
30 degrees	5 lb	8.66 lb
45 degrees	7.07 lb	7.07 lb
60 degrees	8.66 lb	5 lb
90 degrees	10 lb	0 lb
120 degrees	8.66 lb	5 lb

14.

Angle	R	NR
0 degrees	0 lb	50 lb
30 degrees	25 lb	43.4 lb
45 degrees	35.3 lb	35.3 lb
0 degrees	43.3 lb	25 lb
90 degrees	50 lb	0 lb
120 degrees	43.3 lb	25 lb

15. **Muscle**

Muscle	Y	X
VL	139.0 lb	97.5 lb
RF	53 lb	14 lb
VI	150 lb	40 lb
VM	98 lb	-68.8 lb
	440 lb	82.7 lb

a. 454.2 lb up and lateral, 9.4 degrees with vertical

b. 74.4 lb laterally, 4.7 degrees below horizontal

c. 20.6 lb medially

d. 24 lb laterally, 2.8 degrees below the horizontal

Suggested Reading List

Abe M, Medina-Martinez RU, Itoh K, Kohno S. Temporomandibular joint loading generated during bilateral static bites at molars and premolars. *Med Biol Eng Comput.* 2006;44:1017-1030.

Ackland DC, Pandy MG. Lines of action and stabilizing potential of the shoulder musculature. *J Anat.* 2009;215:184-197.

Al-Hayani A. The functional anatomy of hip abductors. *Folia Morphol (Warsz).* 2009;68:98-103.

Amis AA, Senavongse W, Bull, AM. Patellofemoral kinematics during knee flexion-extension: an in vitro study. *J Orthop Res.* 2006;24:2201-2211.

An KN, Kaufman KR, Chao EY. Physiological considerations of muscle force through the elbow joint. *J Biomech.* 1989;22:1249-1256.

An KN, Kwak BM, Chao EY, Morrey BF. Determination of muscle and joint forces: a new technique to solve the indeterminate problem. *J Biomech Eng.* 1984;106:364-367.

Basciftci FA, Korkmaz HH, Usumez S, Eraslan O. Biomechanical evaluation of chincup treatment with various force vectors. *Am J Orthod Dentofacial Orthop.* 2008;134:773-781.

Elias JJ, Cech JA, Weinstein DM, Cosgrea AJ. Reducing the lateral force acting on the patella does not consistently decrease patellofemoral pressures. *Am J Sports Med.* 2004;32:1202-1208.

Elias JJ, Cosgarea AJ. Computational modeling: an alternative approach for investigating patellofemoral mechanics. *Sports Med Arthrosc.* 2007;15:89-94.

Elias JJ, Wilson DR, Adamson R, Cosgarea AJ. Evaluation of a computational model used to predict the patellofemoral contact pressure distribution. *J Biomech.* 2004;37:295-302.

Fagg AH, Shah A, Barto AG. A computational model of muscle recruitment for wrist movements. *J Neurophysiol.* 2002;88:3348-3358.

Flanders M, Soechting JF. Arm muscle activation for static forces in three-dimensional space. *J Neurophysiol.* 1990;64:1818-1837.

Gao F, Latash ML, Zatsiorsky VM. Control of finger force direction in the flexion-extension plane. *Exp Brain Res.* 2005;161:307-315.

Gottschalk F, Kourosh S, Leveau B. The functional anatomy of tensor fasciae latae and gluteus medius and minimus. *J Anat.* 1989;166:179-189.

Hansen ML, Otis JC, Johnson JS, Cordasco FA, Craig EV, Warren RF. Biomechanics of massive rotator cuff tears: implications for treatment. *J Bone Joint Surg Am.* 2008;90:316-325.

Harms MC, Bader DL. Variability of forces applied by experienced therapists during spinal mobilization. *Clin Biomech (Bristol, Avon).* 1997;12:393-399.

Herrington L, Nester C. Q-angle undervalued? The relationship between Q-angle and medio-lateral position of the patella. *Clin Biomech (Bristol, Avon).* 2004;19:1070-1073.

Hoffman DS, Strick PL. Step-tracking movements of the wrist. IV. Muscle activity associated with movements in different directions. *J Neurophysiol.* 1999;81:319-333.

Inman VT. Functional aspects of the abductor muscles of the hip. *J Bone Joint Surg.* 1947;29:607-619.

Kingma I, Staudenmann D, van Dieen JH. Trunk muscle activation and associated lumbar spine joint shear forces under different levels of external forward force applied to the trunk. *J Electromyogr Kinesiol.* 2007;17:14-24.

Kluemper GT, Spalding PM. Realities of craniofacial growth modification. *Atlas Oral Maxillofac Surg Clin North Am.* 2001;9:23-51.

Konrad GG, Jolly JT, Labriola JE, McMahon PJ, Debski RE. Thoracohumeral muscle activity alters glenohumeral joint biomechanics during active abduction. *J Orthop Res.* 2006;24:748-756.

Kursa K, Lattanza L, Diao E, Rempel D. In vivo flexor tendon forces increase with finger and wrist flexion during active finger flexion and extension. *J Orthop Res.* 2006;24:763-769.

Labriola JE, Lee TQ, Debski RE, McMahon PJ. Stability and instability of the glenohumeral joint: the role of shoulder muscles. *J Shoulder Elbow Surg.* 2005;14:32S-38S.

Majima M, Horii E, Matsuki H, Hirata H, Genda E. Load transmission through the wrist in the extended position. *J Hand Surg Am.* 2008;33:182-188.

Mizuno Y, Kumagai M, Mattessich SM, et al. Q-angle influences tibiofemoral and patellofemoral kinematics. *J Orthop Res.* 2001;19:834-840.

Nozaki D, Nakazawa K, Akai M. Muscle activity determined by cosine tuning with a nontrivial preferred direction during isometric force exertion by lower limb. *J Neurophysiol.* 2005;93:2614-2624.

Oizumi N, Tadano S, Narita Y, Suenaga N, Iwasaki N, Minami A. Numerical analysis of cooperative abduction muscle forces in a human shoulder joint. *J Shoulder Elbow Surg.* 2006;15:331-338.

Pataky TC, Latash ML, Zatsiorsky VM. Prehension synergies during nonvertical grasping, I: experimental observations. *Biol Cybern.* 2004;91:148-158.

Pataky TC, Latash ML, Zatsiorsky VM. Prehension synergies during nonvertical grasping, II: Modeling and optimization. *Biol Cybern.* 2004;91:231-242.

Pearlman JL, Roach SS, Valero-Cuevas FJ. The fundamental thumb-tip force vectors produced by the muscles of the thumb. *J Orthop Res.* 2004;22:306-312.

Sharkey NA, Marder RA. The rotator cuff opposes superior translation of the humeral head. *Am J Sports Med.* 1995;23:270-275.

Snodgrass SJ, Rivett DA, Robertson VJ. Manual forces applied during posterior-to-anterior spinal mobilization: a review of the evidence. *J Manipulative Physiol Ther.* 2006;29:316-329.

Snodgrass SJ, Rivett DA, Robertson VJ, Stojanovski E. Forces applied to the cervical spine during posteroanterior mobilization. *J Manipulative Physiol Ther.* 2009;32:72-83.

Staudenmann D, Potvin JR, Kingma I, Stegeman DF, van Dieen JH. Effects of EMG processing on biomechanical models of muscle joint systems: sensitivity of trunk muscle moments, spinal forces, and stability. *J Biomech.* 2007;40:900-909.

Ueki K, Nakagawa K, Takatsuka S, Yamamoto E, Laskin DM. Comparison of the stress direction on the TMJ in patients with class I, II, and III skeletal relationships. *Orthod Craniofac Res.* 2008;11:43-50.

Valero-Cuevas FJ, Johanson ME, Towles JD. Towards a realistic biomechanical model of the thumb: the choice of kinematic description may be more critical than the solution method or the variability/uncertainty of musculoskeletal parameters. *J Biomech.* 2003;36:1019-1030.

van Eijden TM, Kouwenhoven E, Verburg J, Weijs WA. A mathematical model of the patellofemoral joint. *J Biomech.* 1986;19:219-229.

Yanagawa T, Goodwin CJ, Shelburne KB, Giphart JE, Torry MR, Pandy MG. Contributions of the individual muscles of the shoulder to glenohumeral joint stability during abduction. *J Biomech Eng.* 2008;130:021024.

Zatsiorsky VM, Latash ML. Prehension synergies. *Exerc Sport Sci Rev.* 2004;32:75-80.

chapter 4

Equilibrium

LeVeau BF.
*Biomechanics of Human Motion: Basics and
Beyond for the Health Professions* (pp 71-98).

Objectives
1. Explain the 2 conditions of equilibrium.
2. Draw examples of various combinations of forces acting on a static object.
3. Differentiate between a fixed and a moveable pulley.
4. Differentiate among the 3 classes of levers.
5. Provide examples of levers in the body, in clinical use, and in everyday activities.
6. Solve problems using the 2 conditions of equilibrium.

Static Equilibrium

Part of Newton's First Law states that an object at rest tends to remain at rest unless acted upon by external forces. This is the basis of static equilibrium. Statics is the study of objects at rest. Remember that a force is a push or pull that tends to cause a body to change its state of motion. In order for a body to be in a state of equilibrium, the sum of the forces and torques acting on the body must equal zero. The 2 conditions of static equilibrium are presented in this section.

First Condition of Equilibrium

The first condition of equilibrium states that the sum of the forces acting on an object equals zero ($\Sigma F = 0$). This equation is often used to determine the magnitude, line of application, and direction of the forces acting on an object. If the forces are collinear or concurrent, the graphic and mathematical solutions are similar to the processes of resolution and composition. In the graphical method for the composition of 2 concurrent forces (Figure 4-1A), the resultant has its tail at the point of origin and its head located at the head of the last force drawn (Figure 4-1B). In the first condition of equilibrium, this resultant is replaced by a vector called the equilibrant. The equilibrant is equal in magnitude and has the same line of application, but is opposite in direction from the resultant. To graphically draw the equilibrant, its tail is placed at the head of the last force drawn, and its head is at the point of origin (Figure 4-1C). If the arrows are placed head to tail beginning and ending at the graphic point of origin, the polygon is completely closed, and the sum of the forces is zero.

LeVeau BF.
*Biomechanics of Human Motion: Basics and
Beyond for the Health Professions* (pp 71-98).
© 2011 SLACK Incorporated

Figure 4-1. Graphical representation of 2 concurrent forces with resultant and equilibrant.

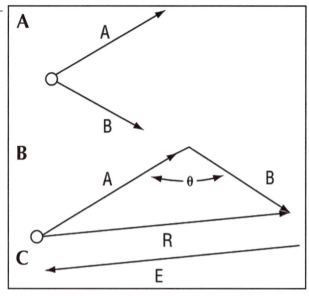

In the previous chapter, the linear force system was introduced. All of the forces lie on the same line (collinear) and in the same plane (coplanar). The problem of a vertical weight rack holding 2 dumbbells, one weighing 10 lb and the other 5 lb, was solved. Their resultant weight was determined to be 15 lb pulling downward. How much force was the weight rack using to maintain the static position of the weights? The answer for equilibrium is the equilibrant or the force equal in magnitude, along the same line of application, but opposite in direction (Figure 4-2). The equilibrant is 15 lb vertically acting upward. The equilibrant in the concurrent system is also equal in magnitude, along the same line of application, but opposite in direction compared to the resultant.

To mathematically solve equilibrium problems, a diagram with all forces and distances should be drawn to scale. Such a diagram is called a free body diagram. For mathematical solutions of the first condition of equilibrium, all forces up and to the right are considered positive, and all forces down and to the left are considered negative. This convention for the signs allows us to determine the magnitude, line of application, and direction from the mathematical solution.

EXAMPLES

Suppose a box resting on a table applies a 20-lb force downward on the table (Figure 4-3). According to Newton's Third Law (the law of reaction), an equal force is acting upon the box. The first law of equilibrium can confirm this law as follows.

$$\Sigma F = 0$$
$$\Sigma F = (\text{-20 lb}) + R = 0$$
$$\text{-20 lb} + R = 0$$
$$R = 20 \text{ lb}$$

The mathematical solution of the problem shows that the reaction force is 20 lb upward.

A tug-of-war at a picnic reveals a similar solution horizontally (Figure 4-4). Suppose that team A is composed of 2 competitors who can pull with 100 lb (A1) and 125 lb (A2) to the left. Team B has 3 members with B1 pulling 45 lb and B2 pulling 50 lb to the right. How much force does member B3 need to pull to keep team B from losing?

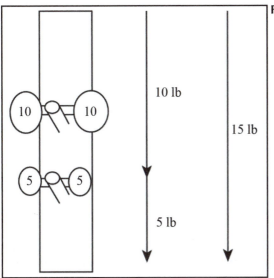

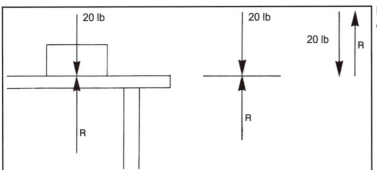

Figure 4-2. Linear force system of weights on a rack.

Figure 4-3. Linear force system of a box on a table.

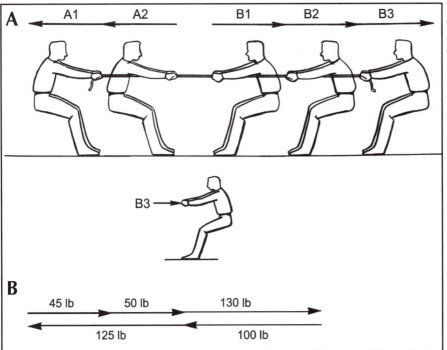

Figure 4-4. Tug-of-war represents a horizontal linear system.

The mathematical solution to this problem is as follows.

$$\Sigma F = 0$$
$$[(45\ lb) + (50\ lb) + (B3)] + [(-100\ lb) + (-125\ lb)] = 0$$
$$[95\ lb + B3] - [225\ lb] = 0$$
$$B3 - 130\ lb = 0$$
$$B3 = 130\ lb$$

Team member B3 must pull with 130 lb of force to the right to keep team B from losing.

Figure 4-5 shows an individual holding a 5-lb weight in his hand with his 10 lb upper limb hanging vertically with 0 degrees of abduction. The supraspinatus muscle is applying a force of 20 lb horizontally to the humerus. What is the joint reaction force of the glenoid fossa on the head of the humerus?

This problem has forces acting up and down and to the right and left. Thus, we need to graph the forces (Figure 4-5A) to visualize the vertical forces (y direction) and the horizontal forces (x direction).

$$\Sigma F_y = 0$$
$$(-5\ lb) + (-10\ lb) + F = 0$$
$$(-15\ lb) + F = 0$$
$$F = 15\ lb$$
$$\Sigma F_x = 0$$
$$(-20\ lb) + F = 0$$
$$F = 20\ lb$$
$$R^2 = F_y^2 + F_x^2 - 2F_yF_x\cos\Theta$$
$$R^2 = (20\ lb)^2 + (15\ lb)^2 - (2)(20\ lb)(15\ lb)(\cos 90\ degrees)$$
$$R^2 = 400\ lb + 225\ lb + 0\ lb$$
$$R^2 = 625\ lb$$
$$R = 25\ lb$$
$$\frac{F_x}{F_y} = \tan\Theta$$
$$\frac{15\ lb}{20\ lb} = \tan\Theta$$
$$0.75 = \tan\Theta$$
$$\theta = 36.87\ degrees$$

The reaction force in the glenohumeral joint is 25 lb acting at a 36.87 degrees angle with the horizontal.

PULLEYS

Pulleys are used to change the line of application of force or to decrease the magnitude of force needed to move a load. The 2 basic types of pulleys are the fixed pulley and the moveable pulley (Figure 4-6).

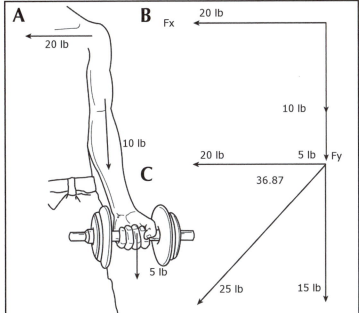

Figure 4-5. Concurrent force system acting on the shoulder.

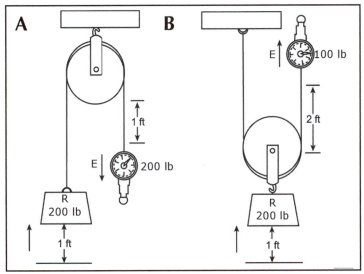

Figure 4-6. Pulleys representing parallel force systems. (A) Fixed pulley. (B) Moveable pulley.

Fixed Pulley

A pulley that is attached to a stationary support is considered a fixed pulley (Figure 4-6A). The fixed pulley is used to change the line of application and the direction of the force. Consider a cord attached to a 50-lb object (Figure 4-7). An individual could lift the object by pulling up with 50 lb of force on the cord. By using a fixed pulley, the individual can pull down with 50 lb of force on the cord to lift the object. Thus, the individual can use body weight (gravitational force) to help lift the object instead of only muscular force. Note that in either situation (with a frictionless pulley), the cord is always transmitting the load provided by the attached object. The fixed pulley does not decrease the magnitude of force needed to move the object. It does allow an individual to apply force to an object in a more favorable position. Often, 2 or more fixed pulleys may be used to direct the force.

Figure 4-7. Fixed pulley used to change the line of application and direction of force.

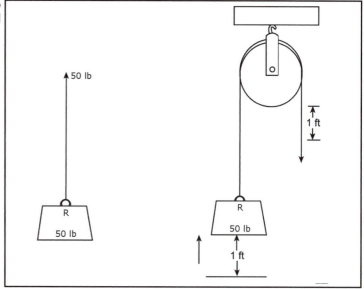

Example: Suppose a therapist is to provide cervical traction to a client (Figure 4-8). The weight of the head is 10 lb, and the therapist wants to apply 15 lb of force to the soft tissues of the posterior cervical area. The traction setup has the harness cord pulling vertically. What magnitude of force needs to be applied to the cord?

$$\Sigma F_y = 0$$
$$(-10 \text{ lb}) + (-15 \text{ lb}) + F_y = 0$$
$$(-25 \text{ lb}) + F_y = 0$$
$$F_y = 25 \text{ lb}$$

Suppose that the traction setup has the harness cord making a 20-degree angle with the vertical to provide some neck flexion (Figure 4-9). What force must be applied to the cord in this situation?

$$F_y = 25 \text{ lb}$$
$$\frac{F_y}{F} = \cos 20 \text{ degrees}$$
$$\frac{F_y}{\cos 20 \text{ degrees}} = F$$
$$\frac{25 \text{ lb}}{0.866} = F$$
$$F = 26.6 \text{ lb}$$

The force necessary to obtain 15 lb of tension in the soft tissues is 26.6 lb. Note that, as the cord passes around a pulley, a force is applied to the pulley and the pulley attachment. For this pulley system acting with a 20-degree angle, a horizontal as well as a vertical force is acting on the pulley. In this setup, how much force is applied to the fixed pulley?

This problem can be solved in 2 ways.

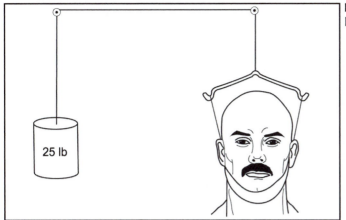

Figure 4-8. Traction using a fixed pulley.

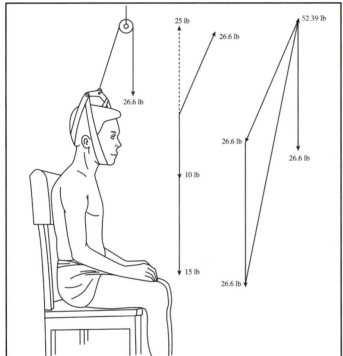

Figure 4-9. Traction using a fixed pulley at 20 degrees.

First, we know that the 2 forces acting on the pulley are equal, both 26.6 lb. With the 2 forces being equal, the angle between them of 20 degrees is bisected to form two 10-degree angles. The solution should use the resolution of forces as follows.

$$F^2 = A^2 + B^2 - 2AB\cos\Theta$$

$$F^2 = (26.6 \text{ lb})^2 + (26.6 \text{ lb})^2 - (2)(26.6 \text{ lb})(26.6 \text{ lb})(\cos 160 \text{ degrees})$$

$$F^2 = 707.56 \text{ lb} + 707.56 \text{ lb} - (2)(26.6 \text{ lb})(26.6 \text{ lb})(-0.940)$$

$$F^2 = 707.56 \text{ lb} + 707.56 \text{ lb} + 1330.2$$

$$F^2 = 2745.33 \text{ lb}$$

$$F = 52.39 \text{ lb}$$

Thus, the load on the pulley support is 52.39 lb.

The second solution uses the first condition of equilibrium and the resolution of forces as follows.

$$\Sigma F_y = 0$$

$$(-25 \text{ lb}) + (-26.6 \text{ lb}) + F = 0$$

$$(-51.6 \text{ lb}) + F = 0$$

$$F_y = 51.6 \text{ lb}$$

$$\Sigma F_x = 0$$

$$(25 \sin 20 \text{ degrees}) + F_x = 0$$

$$(25 \times 0.342) + F_x = 0$$

$$8.55 + F_x = 0$$

$$F_x = -8.55 \text{ lb}$$

$$F^2 = F_y{}^2 + F_x{}^2 - 2F_yF_x\cos\Theta$$

$$F^2 = (51.6 \text{ lb})^2 + (-8.55 \text{ lb})^2 - (2)(51.5 \text{ lb})(-8.55 \text{ lb})(\cos 90 \text{ degrees})$$

$$F^2 = 2662.56 \text{ lb} + 73.1 \text{ lb} + 0 \text{ lb}$$

$$F^2 = 2735.66 \text{ lb}$$

$$F = 52.3 \text{ lb}$$

$$\tan \Theta = \frac{F_x}{F_y}$$

$$\tan \Theta = \frac{-8.55 \text{ lb}}{51.6 \text{ lb}}$$

$$\tan \Theta = 0.1657$$

$$\Theta = 9.4 \text{ degrees with the vertical}$$

The magnitude of force found by the 2 solutions are within 0.09 lb of each other, and the line of application is within 0.6 degrees, which can be accounted for by rounding procedures. Note that the force on the pulley is often greater than the force in the cord.

Many examples of the fixed pulley are found in the body. For example, a bony prominence, such as the lateral malleolus, serves as a pulley around which the tendon acts as the cord of the pulley system (Figure 4-10). The femoral condyles act as a pulley with the quadriceps tendon and patella as the cord (Figure 4-11). Many exercise devices use more than one pulley to direct the load of gravity pulley on a weight stack (Figures 4-12, 4-13, and 4-14). Knowing the force on the pulley can be very important. For example, the force on the body pulleys, such as on the femoral condyles, may lead to chondromalacia patella.

Moveable Pulley

A moveable pulley is generally used to decrease the force needed to move the object. The moveable pulley is generally not designed to change the line of application or direction of the force. One end of the cord in a moveable pulley system is fixed, while a force is applied to the other end. The load is attached to a pulley that is allowed to move (Figure 4-15). Therefore, the moveable pulley system with a load of 20 lb and 2 vertical cords would have the force through the cord as follows. Remember that the force in the cord is always the same value in a frictionless pulley system.

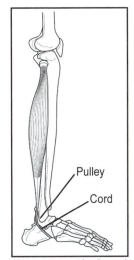

Figure 4-10. The lateral malleolus as a pulley.

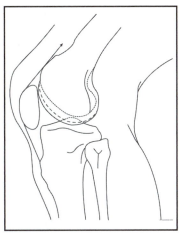

Figure 4-11. Femoral condyles as a pulley.

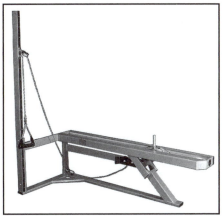

Figure 4-12. Pulleys on the Impulse Inertial Exercise Trainer. (Courtesy of Impulse Training Systems, Newnan, GA.)

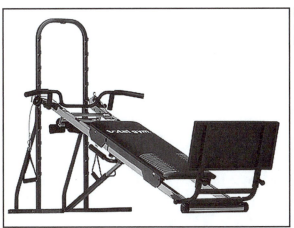

Figure 4-13. Pulleys on the Total Gym. Reprinted with permission from Patterson Medical/ Sammons Preston, Bolingbrook, IL.

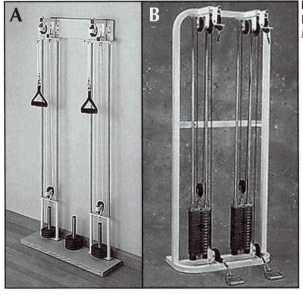

Figure 4-14. Various types of wall pulleys. Reprinted with permission from Patterson Medical/Sammons Preston, Bolingbrook, IL.

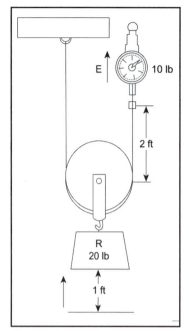

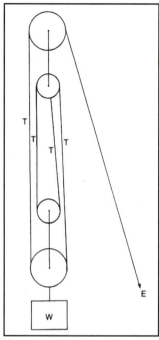

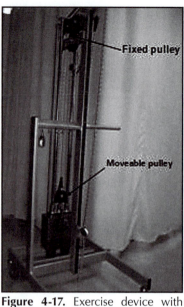

Figure 4-17. Exercise device with fixed and moveable pulleys.

Figure 4-15. Moveable pulley used to decrease the force needed to move an object by increasing the mechanical advantage.

Figure 4-16. Moveable pulley system with 4 supporting strands.

$$\Sigma F_y = 0$$
$$F_1 + F_2 + (\text{-20 lb}) = 0$$
$$F_1 = F_2 = F$$
$$2F + (\text{-20 lb}) = 0$$
$$2F = 20 \text{ lb}$$
$$F = 10 \text{ lb}$$

The force on the cord is 10 lb or half of the load. Disadvantages of the moveable pulley system are that the applied force must move twice as far as the load, and the applied force moves twice as fast as the load. The mechanical advantage of a pulley system can be determined by the number of supporting strands of the cord or the load divided by the force applied to the cord. The mechanical advantage of the worked example is 2.

Fixed and moveable pulleys can be used in combination to change direction and increase the mechanical advantage (Figure 4-16). Many exercise devices using pulleys have a combination of fixed and moveable pulleys (Figure 4-17).

Second Condition of Equilibrium

In many situations, the acting forces are not concurrent. The forces may be acting in the same plane (coplanar) and parallel to each other. Such a force system, called a parallel force system, is a special case of the general force system. The general force system has forces acting on an object that are neither collinear nor concurrent, and not always parallel. In these situations, the forces tend to cause the object to rotate around a pivot point or axis. For the object to remain at rest without rotating, it must adhere to the second condition of equilibrium.

That is, the sum of the torques acting on an object must equal zero ($\Sigma M = 0$). The moment is the application of a force at a distance from the point of pivot for that object (Figure 4-18). The distance (d) from the point of application of the force to the pivot point can be called the lever arm, or moment arm. Because the force is not acting through the pivot point, it tends to turn the object around this point. To remain in static equilibrium, another moment or moments must tend to turn the object in the opposite direction (Figure 4-19). The directions for moments are not up, down, right, or left, but are clockwise and counterclockwise. Engineers have established the convention for mathematical analysis that counterclockwise moments are positive and clockwise moments are negative. To determine the actual moment applied to an object, the force component (F_r) that is perpendicular to the lever arm must be used (Figure 4-20). Therefore, the definition of a moment is often stated as the force times its perpendicular distance from the axis (torque). The ability to determine force components is essential in order to evaluate the effect of moments on an object.

To determine the magnitude of a moment in some situations, the distance (d_1) measured from the point of rotation (O) perpendicular to the applied force (F) times the applied force may be used instead of the perpendicular force component (F_r) drawn from the point of application times the distance from the point of rotation to the point of application (d) (Figure 4-21).

The following equations will show that either approach will provide the same result.

Component Method	**Lever Method**
Moment = F_r x d	Moment = F x d_1
F_r = (F x cosΘ)	d_1 = (d x cosΘ)
Moment = (F x cosΘ) x d	Moment = F x (d x cosΘ)

Note that the moment determined by either equation has the same factors of F, d, and cosΘ. Why is the angle between the force, F, and the force component, F_r, equal to Θ (Figure 4-22)?

Since the sum of all angles within a triangle is 180 degrees, then

$$\Theta + 90 \text{ degrees} + (\Phi) = 180 \text{ degrees};$$

$$\Phi = 180 \text{ degrees} - 90 \text{ degrees} - \Theta; \text{ and}$$

$$\Phi = 90 \text{ degrees} - \Theta$$

The force component, F_r, is perpendicular or 90 degrees to the lever. Therefore,

$$90 \text{ degrees} - \Phi = \Theta$$

Because a moment is the product of force and lever length, a predictable relationship for lever systems can be determined. If one lever arm is twice as long as a second lever arm, the perpendicular force component applied to the first lever arm must be one-half the magnitude of that applied to the second. The second condition of equilibrium deals with moments or forces and lever arms. Therefore, an understanding of lever systems may be of value.

LEVERS

A lever is defined as a rigid bar that turns around an axis. Levers can provide a mechanical advantage (MA) by requiring less force to move a larger load. To determine the mechanical advantage of a lever system, the length of the force arm, d_f, is divided by the length of the load arm d_1 (Figure 4-23), or

$$MA = \frac{d_f}{d_1}$$

Levers can also increase the load's speed and distance moved compared to the speed and distance moved for the force. See Table 4-1 for a comparison of the 3 classes of levers.

Figure 4-18. Application of force (F) at a distance (d) from an axis. The moment = F x d.

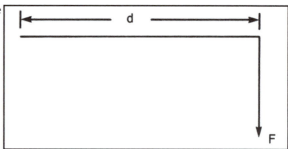

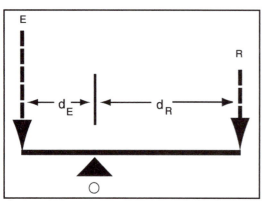

Figure 4-19. Two moments are needed to keep the rotation in equilibrium.

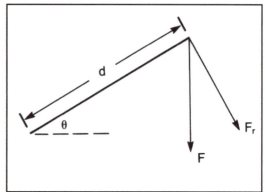

Figure 4-20. The perpendicular force component (F_r) is used to determine the moment.

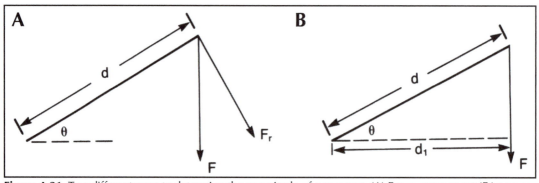

Figure 4-21. Two different ways to determine the magnitude of a moment: (A) Force component (F_r) perpendicular to the force arm (d). (B) The force (F) times the distance (d_1) perpendicular to the force.

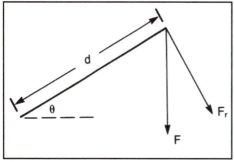

Figure 4-22. The angle of the force component is equal to the angle of the lever with the horizontal.

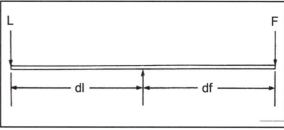

Figure 4-23. The mechanical advantage of the lever is determined by $\frac{d_f}{d_l}$.

TABLE 4-1

Comparison of the Three Classes of Levers

Class of Lever	d_f compared to d_l**	MA	Effect on speed of load	Effect on distance load moves	Examples
First class (FOL)*	d_f equal to d_l	=1	Same speed	Same distance	Seesaw
	d_f longer than d_l	>1	Load slower	Load moves less	Crowbar
	d_f shorter than d_l	<1	Load faster	Load moves more	Triceps on the forearm, gluteus medius on the femur
Second class (OLF)*	d_f longer than d_l	>1	Load slower	Load less	Wheelbarrow, gastrocnemius during heel raise
Third class (OFL)*	d_f shorter than d_l	<1	Load faster	Load greater	Biceps on the forearm, hamstrings on the leg

*Order of the location on the lever: F is the force; O is the axis; L is the load.

**d_f is the length of the force lever to the axis; d_l is the length of the load lever to the axis.

First-Class Levers

Levers are classified simply as first-class, second-class, and third-class. A first-class lever, designated FOL, has the pivot point or axis (O) between the 2 forces, which can be called the force (F) and the load (L) (Figure 4-24A). The force arm (d_f) can be longer, equal to, or shorter than the load arm (d_l). The mechanical advantage can be greater than 1, equal to 1, or less than 1. With this lever, a load can be moved a shorter distance than the force, the same distance as the force, or a greater distance than the force. The load may move slower than the force, equal speed as the force, or faster than the force. If the point of application for the effort is placed 4 times the distance from the axis as the distance for the point of application for the load, the effort will need only one-fourth the magnitude of force to hold the load (Figure 4-25). The mechanical advantage of the lever will be 4. One of the forces will tend to cause the lever to rotate clockwise around the axis, while the other will tend to rotate it counterclockwise. With movement, the force must move 4 times the distance of the load. The point of force application will move 4 times faster than the point of application of the load. The reaction force at the axis must not be forgotten. In this situation, the reaction force on the axis will be 5 times greater than the applied force. The axis reaction force will equal the sum of the applied force plus the load.

To determine the reaction force at the axis in a parallel force system, the first condition of equilibrium is used. In the preceding situation having a load of 400 lb, the applied force would be 100 lb (see Figure 4-25). The force at the axis would be found as follows:

$$\Sigma F_y = 0$$
$$(-400 \text{ lb}) + (-100 \text{ lb}) + A = 0$$
$$-500 + A = 0$$
$$A = 500 \text{ lb}$$

Figure 4-24. Three classes of levers. (A) First class with the axis between the force and load. (B) Second class with the load between the force and axis. (C) Third class with the force between the load and axis.

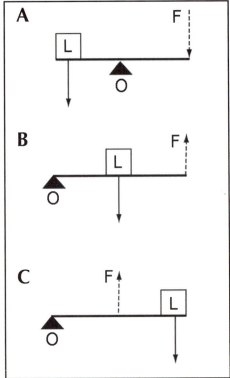

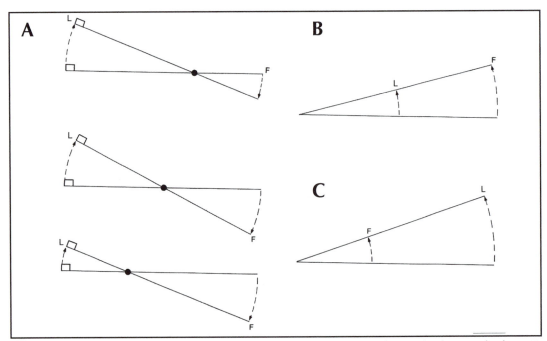

Figure 4-25. With a first class lever having a mechanical advantage greater than 1, the distance the force (F) moves is less than the distance the load (L) moves. With a first class lever having a mechanical advantage equal to 1, the distance the force (F) moves is the same as the distance the load (L) moves. With a first class lever having a mechanical advantage less than 1, the distance the force (F) moves is greater than the distance the load (L) moves. With the second class lever (B), the distance moved and the speed of the applied force (F) will always be greater than that of the load (L). With the third class lever (C), the distance moved and the speed of the applied force (F) will always be less than that of the load (L).

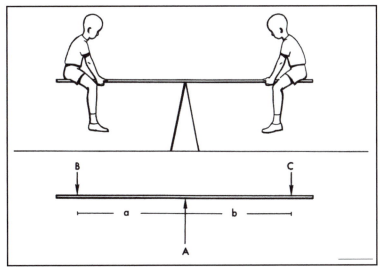

Figure 4-26. The teeter-totter as a first-class lever. Force B tends to turn the lever counterclockwise, while force C tends to turn the lever clockwise. Force A acts upward equal to the combined forces of B + C.

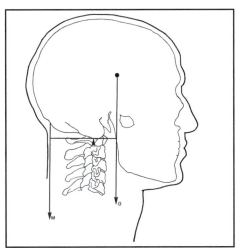

Figure 4-27. The head on the atlas as a first-class lever.

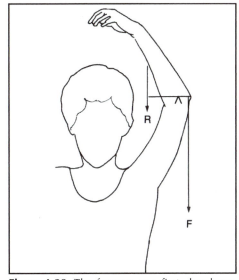

Figure 4-28. The forearm as a first-class lever.

In this situation, the force at the point of rotation is 500 lb acting along a vertical line of application in an upward direction.

Examples of a first-class lever include a teeter-totter or seesaw (Figure 4-26), the head (Figure 4-27), and the forearm (Figure 4-28).

Second-Class Levers

The second-class lever, designated OLF, has the load (L) between the axis (O) and the force (F) (see Figure 4-24B). In this case, the magnitude of the force is always less than the load, and the force lever is always longer than the load arm. Therefore, the mechanical advantage is always greater than 1. The distance moved and the speed of the applied force (F) will always be greater than the load (L) as shown in Figure 4-25B. With only the 3 forces involved, the magnitude of the reaction force at the axis (O) will always be less than that of the load (L). A wheelbarrow is an example of a second-class lever (Figure 4-29).

Figure 4-29. The wheelbarrow as a second-class lever.

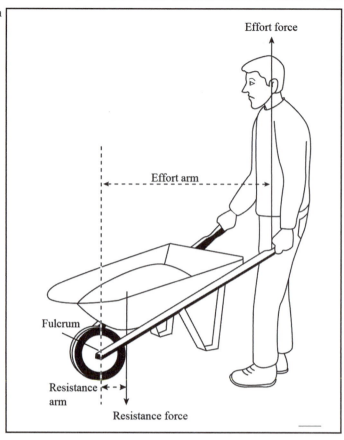

Third-Class Levers

The third-class lever, designated OFL, has the force (F) between the load (L) and the axis (O) (see Figure 4-24C). In this situation, the magnitude of the force is always greater than the load, and the mechanical advantage is always less than 1. However, the load (L) will always move farther and faster than the force (F) as shown in Figure 4-25C. The body is designed with many third-class levers. Such an arrangement works well for throwing a baseball, kicking a football, and holding objects in the hand. With only the 3 forces involved, the magnitude of the reaction force at the axis (O) will be less than that of the applied force (F). The forearm is an example of a third-class lever (Figure 4-30).

Levers are often considered to be straight rigid bars. However, a lever can be bent into any configuration such as a hammer pulling a nail (Figure 4-31) or the gluteus medius pulling on the femur (Figure 4-32). A wheel and axle or crank and axle also act like a lever with continuous rotation (Figure 4-33), such as a screwdriver (Figure 4-34) or the teres minor rotating the humerus (Figure 4-35).

Knowledge of the specific classification of a lever system is not essential but it helps to understand the relationships of forces, lever arms, and mechanical advantage. A situation involving levers will provide information about lever lengths and at least one force (often the load). The most basic situation involves 3 parallel forces with their points of application and each force known, but the magnitude of only one force known.

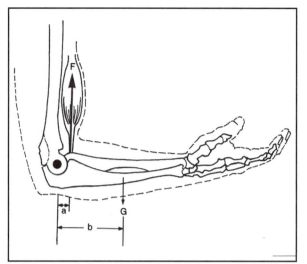

Figure 4-30. The forearm as a third-class lever.

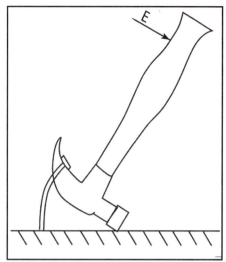

Figure 4-31. The hammer as a bent lever.

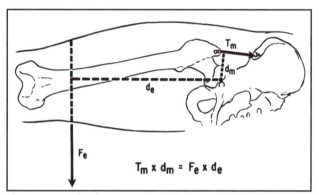

Figure 4-32. The femur as a bent lever.

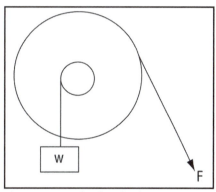

Figure 4-33. Wheel and axle as a continuous lever.

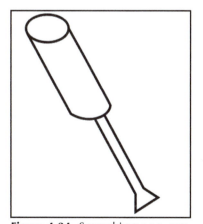

Figure 4-34. Screwdriver as a continuous lever.

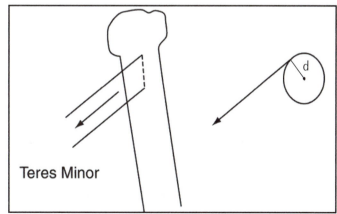

Figure 4-35. Teres minor acting on the humerus as a continuous lever.

EXAMPLES

Parallel Systems of Forces

An individual is holding the forearm in a horizontal position (Figure 4-36). The forearm and hand weigh 10 lb with their combined center of mass located 6 in from the elbow joint. The elbow flexor muscles considered as a group attach 2 in from the elbow joint. What is the elbow flexor muscle force needed to maintain this position? What is the joint reaction force at the elbow? To solve this problem, a figure (free body diagram) should be drawn with all of the forces and lengths shown (Figure 4-37). The second condition of equilibrium equation ($\Sigma M = 0$) should first be used to find the solution.

$$\Sigma M = 0$$

joint reaction moment + muscle moment + limb weight moment = 0

$$(Jdj) + (Mdm) + (Wdw) = 0$$

This problem has 2 unknown values, but only one equation. However, if the joint is taken as the axis with its lever length (dj) equal to zero, the joint moment (Jdj) becomes zero.

$$(J \times 0 \text{ in}) + (M \times 2 \text{ in}) + (10 \text{ lb} \times 6 \text{ in}) = 0$$

$$0 + (M \times 2 \text{ in}) + (60 \text{ in} \bullet \text{lb}) = 0$$

$$M \times 2 \text{ in} = 60 \text{ in} \bullet \text{lb}$$

$$M = \frac{60 \text{ in} \bullet \text{lb}}{2 \text{ in}}$$

$$M = 30 \text{ lb}$$

Therefore, the muscle force needed to maintain the forearm and hand in a horizontal position is 30 lb. Now, the joint force can be determined using the first condition of equilibrium equation $\Sigma F = 0$. In this situation, all of the forces are parallel, acting vertically along the y-coordinate. No horizontal force or F_x is involved. Therefore,

$$\Sigma F_y = 0$$

$$J_y + M_y + W_y = 0$$

$$J_y + 30 \text{ lb} + (-10 \text{ lb}) = 0$$

$$J_y + 20 \text{ lb} = 0$$

$$J_y = -20 \text{ lb}$$

The joint reaction force in this situation is 20 lb acting downward.

Suppose the individual added a load of 20 lb to the hand 15 in from the elbow joint (Figure 4-38). What is the muscle force and joint reaction force in this situation? The solution to the problem is similar to the previous one except that a moment for the load is added to the equation to get the following:

$$\Sigma M = 0$$

joint reaction moment + muscle moment + limb weight moment + load moment = 0

$$(Jdj) + (Mdm) + (Wdw) + (Ldl) = 0$$

$$(J \times 0 \text{ in}) + (M \times 2 \text{ in}) + (10 \text{ lb} \times 6 \text{ in}) + (20 \text{ lb} \times 15 \text{ in}) = 0$$

$$0 + (M \times 2 \text{ in}) + (60 \text{ in} \bullet \text{lb}) + (300 \text{ in} \bullet \text{lb}) = 0$$

$$M \times 2 \text{ in} = 360 \text{ in} \bullet \text{lb}$$

$$M = \frac{360 \text{ in} \bullet \text{lb}}{2 \text{ in}}$$

$$M = 180 \text{ lb}$$

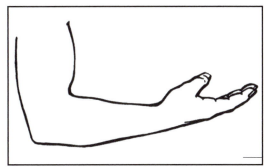

Figure 4-36. Forearm in a horizontal position.

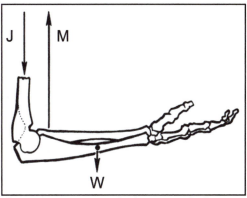

Figure 4-37. Forces on the forearm in the horizontal position.

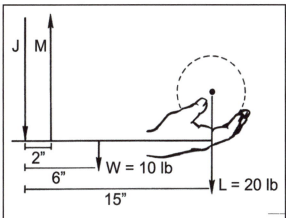

Figure 4-38. Forces on the forearm in the horizontal position while holding a load.

Therefore, the muscle force needed to maintain the forearm and hand in a horizontal position is 180 lb, which is much greater than without a load. Now, with the addition of the load, the joint force can be determined using the first condition of equilibrium equation.

$$\Sigma F_y = 0$$
$$J_y + M_y + W_y + L_y = 0$$
$$J_y + 180 \text{ lb} + (\text{-}10 \text{ lb}) + (\text{-}20 \text{ lb}) = 0$$
$$J_y + 150 \text{ lb} = 0$$
$$J_y = \text{-}150 \text{ lb}$$

The joint reaction force increases greatly in magnitude with the load added.

General Systems of Forces

Suppose the upper limb is flexed 60 degrees at the shoulder from the anatomical position and the hand is holding a 20 lb load 28 in from the shoulder joint (Figure 4-39). The weight of the upper limb is 12 lb with its center of mass 14 in from the shoulder joint. The deltoid muscle has a 15-degree line of application with the upper limb with a point of application 6 in from the shoulder joint. What are the muscle and joint forces in this situation?

Figure 4-39. An example of the general force system. Shoulder flexion.

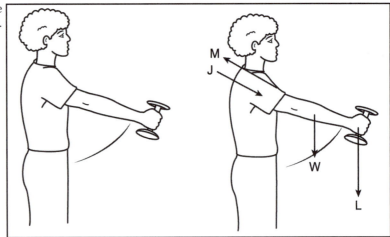

For this problem, the figure should be drawn with the rotatory and non-rotatory force components included. The upper limb should be considered the x-axis with the y-axis perpendicular to it. Thus, the rotatory forces will be parallel to the y-axis and perpendicular to the x-axis, while the non-rotatory forces will be parallel to the x-axis. The point of rotation should be set at the joint (J) to eliminate the joint reaction force moment. The second condition of equilibrium ($\Sigma M = 0$) is used to determine the muscle force. Note that the rotatory component for the deltoid muscle is M times the sin 15 degrees, for the weight force is the weight times the sin 60 degrees (cos 30 degrees), and for the load force is the load times the sin 60 degrees (cos 30 degrees).

$$\Sigma M = 0$$

joint reaction moment + muscle moment + limb weight moment + load moment = 0

$$(Jdj) + (Mydm) + (Wydw) + (Lydl) = 0$$

$$(J \times 0) + [(M \times \sin 15 \text{ degrees}) \times 6 \text{ in}] + [(12 \text{ lb} \times \sin 60 \text{ degrees}) \times 14 \text{ in}] +$$
$$[(20 \text{ lb} \times \sin 60 \text{ degrees}) \times 28 \text{ in}] = 0$$

$$(M \times 0.259 \times 6 \text{ in}) + (12 \text{ lb} \times 0.866 \times 14 \text{ in}) + (20 \text{ lb} \times 0.866 * 28 \text{ in}) = 0$$

$$(M \times 1.55 \text{ in}) + (145.49 \text{ in} \bullet \text{lb}) + (484.97 \text{ in} \bullet \text{lb}) = 0$$

$$M \times 1.55 \text{ in} = 630.46 \text{ in} \bullet \text{lb}$$

$$M = \frac{630.46 \text{ in} \bullet \text{lb}}{1.55 \text{ in}}$$

$$M = 406.7 \text{ lb}$$

$$\Sigma F_y = 0$$

$$J_y + M_y + W_y + L_y = 0$$

$$J_y + (406.7 \times \sin 15 \text{ degrees}) + (-12 \text{ lb} \times \sin 60 \text{ degrees}) + (-20 \text{ lb} \times \sin 60 \text{ degrees}) = 0$$

$$J_y + (105.27 \text{ lb}) - (10.39 \text{ lb}) - (17.32 \text{ lb}) = 0$$

$$J_y = -77.56 \text{ lb}$$

$$\Sigma F_x = 0$$

$$J_x + M_x + W_x + L_x = 0$$

$$J_x + (406.7 \times \cos 15 \text{ degrees}) + (-12 \text{ lb} \times \cos 60 \text{ degrees}) + (-20 \text{ lb} \times \cos 60 \text{ degrees}) = 0$$

$$J_x + (-392.8 \text{ lb}) + (6 \text{ lb}) + (10 \text{ lb}) = 0$$

$$J_x = 376.8 \text{ lb}$$

$$\frac{F_x}{F_y} = \tan\Theta$$

$$\frac{77.56 \text{ lb}}{376.8 \text{ lb}} = \tan\Theta$$

$$0.2058 = \tan\Theta$$

$$\theta = 11.6 \text{ degrees with the x-axis (upper limb)}$$

$$J^2 = Jy^2 + Jx^2 - (2J_yJ_x\cos\Theta)$$

$$J^2 = (77.56 \text{ lb})^2 + (376.8 \text{ lb})^2 - [(2)(77.56 \text{ lb})(376.8 \text{ lb})(\cos 90 \text{ degrees})]$$

$$J^2 = 6015.55 \text{ lb} + 141978.24 \text{ lb} + 0 \text{ lb}$$

$$J^2 = 147993.8 \text{ lb}$$

$$J = 384.7 \text{ lb}$$

The magnitude of muscle force to hold the weighted limb in this position is 406.7 lb. The reaction force at the joint is 384.7 lb acting at an angle of 11.6 degrees with the upper limb.

Human Body Examples

The human body is composed of many lever arm situations, and many lever situations are imposed upon the body. The pull by the gluteus medius muscle acting on the pelvis is an example of a first-class lever (Figure 4-40), the gastrocnemius lifting the heel is an example of a second-class lever (Figure 4-41), and the pull by the hamstring muscles is an example of a third-class lever (Figure 4-42).

Many examples to determine individual muscle forces and moments have been presented and based upon data derived from body segment and position estimates or inverse dynamics discussed in Chapter 6. In recent years, more sophisticated models have been considered to make the calculations more accurate and clinically relevant. The present models provide insight into what is happening during the posture or activity, but are only estimates of what is actually happening. These estimates, however, can give the practitioner an idea about concerns such as the effectiveness of an exercise or treatment, the cause of an injury, or the design of a splint or exercise device. The determination of the forces (although estimates) can help one understand the forces and moments and can be done quickly and easily.

The effect of a load or muscle force on any lever system can be easily determined by following a few steps:

- Draw a free body diagram of the situation being analyzed
- Establish all x and y components of forces perpendicular and parallel to the body part
- Choose the coordinate axes (x and y) and moment center (at point of unknown force)
- If necessary, divide the line diagram into isolated sections
- Solve for unknown forces using the second condition of equilibrium
- Solve for the remaining unknown force using the first condition of equilibrium equation, cosine law, and trigonometric functions

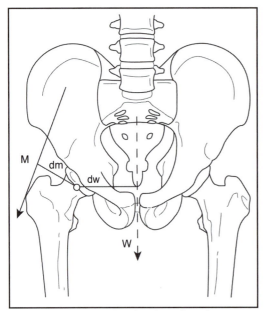

Figure 4-40. Example of a first-class lever: Hip moments during gait. W is the superincumbent weight, and M is the abductor muscle force.

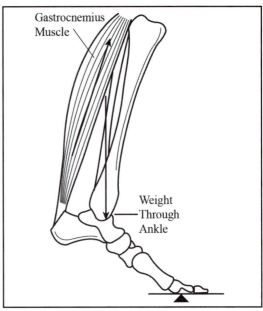

Figure 4-41. Example of a second-class lever: Gastrocnemius acting on the foot. R is the ground reaction force at the axis of the lever system that is equal to the body weight (W) as an individual stands on tiptoes, L is the load passing through the talocural joint, and M is the muscle force lifting the calcaneus off the ground.

Figure 4-42. Example of a third-class lever: Hamstrings acting on the leg. M is the muscle force, and L is the load, both acting around the axis.

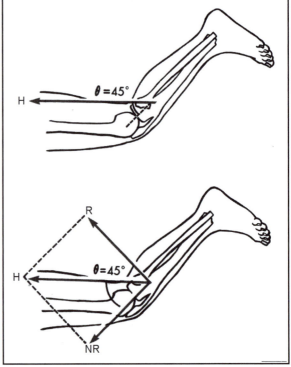

Activities

1. Explain the difference between the first and the second conditions of equilibrium.

2. Why are no moments of force present if the forces are concurrent?

3. Draw and explain the forces involved for the following situations:
   a. Sitting with knee extension with cuff weight
   b. Hip during stance phase of gait (frontal plane)
   c. Sidelying hip abduction
   d. Shoulder flexion with dumbbell
   e. Elbow extension with dumbbell
   f. Back for 2 methods of lifting a box
   g. Elbow flexion with dumbbell

4. Which muscle attachment has a greater effect in producing rotatory motion—one that pulls perpendicular to the bone or one that pulls parallel to the bone?

5. Differentiate between a fixed pulley and a moveable pulley.

6. Explain the difference between sitting and the supine position in applying cervical traction.

7. Explain how changing the position of the body part affects the muscle force needed to hold that body part in the final position.

8. Explain how the magnitude, line of application, and direction of muscle force affects the joint reaction force.

9. Compare the advantages and disadvantages of the 3 classes of levers.

10. Compare the moments of an individual performing abdominal curls with the arms at the sides, across the chest, and arms behind the head.

11. Draw and describe the moments involved as an individual does double leg lowering.

12. Solve the problems in Figure 4-43.

13. Suppose that as an individual ascends a step, the quadriceps muscles pull with a combined force of 300 lb on the patella, and the patellar tendon is pulling with 300 lb on the patella. The angle between the muscle and tendon forces is 65 degrees. What is the reaction force by the femoral condyles on the patella?

14. Two therapists wish to transfer a 160-lb patient from a wheelchair. Therapist A lifts at the trunk 8 in posterior to the patient's center of mass. Therapist B lifts at the ankles 26 in from the patient's center of mass. How much weight will each therapist be supporting?

15. A 90-lb boy sits 5 ft from the axis of a teeter-totter facing a 75-lb girl on the other end of the board. How far from the axis must the girl sit to balance the weight of the boy? Where would the girl have to sit if the boy weighed 60 lb?

16. When a 160-lb person stands at the end of a diving board 12 ft from where it is anchored, what moment is exerted about the fixed point of the board?

17. Rhonda is holding a 20-lb dumbbell in her hand 20 in from her shoulder joint. If the deltoid inserts 5 in from the shoulder joint at an angle of 15 degrees, her upper limb weighs 6 lb, and the center of mass of the upper limb is 9 in from the shoulder joint, how much deltoid muscle force is needed to hold the dumbbell at 0 degrees, 30 degrees, 45 degrees, 60 degrees, 90 degrees, and 120 degrees? What is the joint reaction force at each angle?

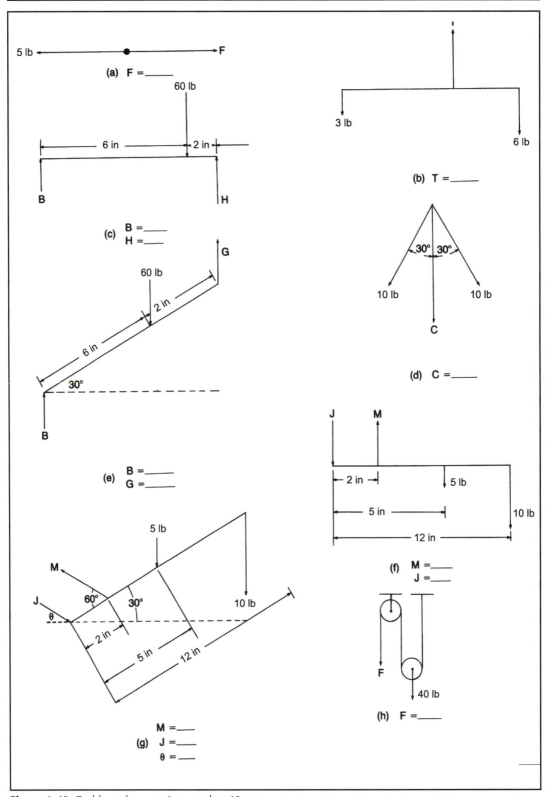

Figure 4-43. Problems for question number 12.

Answers

12.

    a)   5 lb

    b)   9 lb

    c)   15 lb, 45 lb

    d)   17.32 lb

    e)   15 lb, 45 lb

    f)   72.5 lb, -57.5 lb

    g)   72.5 lb, 66.3 lb, 18.8 degrees

    h)   20 lb

13. 506 lb

14. A=122.4 lb, B=37.6 lb

15. A=6 ft, B=4 ft

16. 1920 ft • lb

17.

Degrees	Muscle force	Joint force	Θ
0 degrees	0 lb	26 lb	0 degrees
30 degrees	176	151	12.4 degrees
45 degrees	248.8	226.7	
60 degrees	304.8	283	
90 degrees	351.9	346	
120 degrees	304.8	312.6	

Suggested Reading

Ackland DC, Pak P, Richardson M, Pandy MG. Moment arms of the muscles crossing the anatomical shoulder. *J Anat.* 2008;213:383-390.

Adams CR, Baldwin MA, Laz PJ, Rullkoetter PJ, Langenderfer JE. Effects of rotator cuff tears on muscle moment arms: a computational study. *J Biomech.* 2007;40:3373-3380.

Andersen LL, Nielsen PK, Sogaard K, Andersen CH, Skotte J, Sjogaard G. Torque-EMG-velocity relationship in female workers with chronic neck muscle pain. *J Biomech.* 2008;41:2029-2035.

Arampatzis A, Karamanidis K, De Monte G, Stafilidis S, Morey-Klapsing G, Bruggemann GP. Differences between measured and resultant joint moments during voluntary and artificially elicited isometric knee extension contractions. *Clin Biomech (Bristol, Avon).* 2004;19:277-283.

Arjmand N, Shirazi-Adl A. Model and in vivo studies on human trunk load partitioning and stability in isometric forward flexions. *J Biomech.* 2006;39:510-521.

Bazrgari B, Shirazi-Adl A, Arjmand N. Analysis of squat and stoop dynamic liftings: muscle forces and internal spinal loads. *Eur Spine J.* 2007;16:687-699.

Bremer AK, Sennwald GR, Favre P, Jacob HA. Moment arms of forearm rotators. *Clin Biomech (Bristol, Avon).* 2006;21:683-691.

Brown SH, McGill SM. Co-activation alters the linear versus non-linear impression of the EMG-torque relationship of trunk muscles. *J Biomech.* 2008;41:491-497.

Browne C, Hermida JC, Bergula A, Colwell CW Jr, D'Lima DD. Patellofemoral forces after total knee arthroplasty: effect of extensor moment arm. *Knee.* 2005;12:81-88.

Calisse J, Rohlmann A, Bergmann G. Estimation of trunk muscle forces using the finite element method and in vivo loads measured by telemeterized internal spinal fixation devices. *J Biomech.* 1999;32:727-731.

Chan GN, Smith AW, Kirtley C, Tsang WW. Changes in knee moments with contralateral versus ipsilateral cane usage in females with knee osteoarthritis. *Clin Biomech (Bristol, Avon)*. 2005;20:396-404.

D'Lima DD, Poole C, Chadha H, Hermida JC, Mahar A, Colwell CW Jr. Quadriceps moment arm and quadriceps forces after total knee arthroplasty. *Clin Orthop Relat Res*. 2001:213-220.

Daggfeldt K, Thorstensson A. The mechanics of back-extensor torque production about the lumbar spine. *J Biomech*. 2003;36:815-825.

DeVita P, Hortobagyi T. Obesity is not associated with increased knee joint torque and power during level walking. *J Biomech*. 2003;36:1355-1362.

Dickerson CR, Martin BJ, Chaffin DB. The relationship between shoulder torques and the perception of muscular effort in loaded reaches. *Ergonomics*. 2006;49:1036-1051.

Doyle JR. Palmar and digital flexor tendon pulleys. *Clin Orthop Relat Res*. 2001:84-96.

Dumas R, Cheze L. 3D inverse dynamics in non-orthonormal segment coordinate system. *Med Biol Eng Comput*. 2007;45:315-322.

El-Rich M, Shirazi-Adl A, Arjmand N. Muscle activity, internal loads, and stability of the human spine in standing postures: combined model and in vivo studies. *Spine (Phila Pa 1976)*. 2004;29:2633-2642.

Elias JJ, Cosgarea AJ. Computational modeling: an alternative approach for investigating patellofemoral mechanics. *Sports Med Arthrosc*. 2007;15:89-94.

Erdemir A, McLean S, Herzog W, van den Bogert AJ. Model-based estimation of muscle forces exerted during movements. *Clin Biomech (Bristol, Avon)*. 2007;22:131-154.

Escamilla RF. Knee biomechanics of the dynamic squat exercise. *Med Sci Sports Exerc*. 2001;33:127-141.

Escamilla RF, Fleisig GS, Lowry TM, Barrentine SW, Andrews JR. A three-dimensional biomechanical analysis of the squat during varying stance widths. *Med Sci Sports Exerc*. 2001;33:984-998.

Favre P, Jacob HA, Gerber C. Changes in shoulder muscle function with humeral position: a graphical description. *J Shoulder Elbow Surg*. 2009;18:114-121.

Favre P, Sheikh R, Fucentese SF, Jacob HA. An algorithm for estimation of shoulder muscle forces for clinical use. *Clin Biomech (Bristol, Avon)*. 2005;20:822-833.

Favre P, Snedeker JG, Gerber C. Numerical modelling of the shoulder for clinical applications. *Philos Transact A Math Phys Eng Sci*. 2009;367:2095-2118.

Ford KR, Myer GD, Brent JL, Hewett TE. Hip and knee extensor moments predict vertical jump height in adolescent girls. *J Strength Cond Res*. 2009;23:1327-1331.

Gatti CJ, Dickerson CR, Chadwick EK, Mell AG, Hughes RE. Comparison of model-predicted and measured moment arms for the rotator cuff muscles. *Clin Biomech (Bristol, Avon)*. 2007;22:639-644.

Glitsch U, Baumann W. The three-dimensional determination of internal loads in the lower extremity. *J Biomech*. 1997;30:1123-1131.

Graichen H, Englmeier KH, Reiser M, Eckstein F. An in vivo technique for determining 3D muscular moment arms in different joint positions and during muscular activation—application to the supraspinatus. *Clin Biomech (Bristol, Avon)*. 2001;16:389-394.

Granata KR, Bennett BC. Low-back biomechanics and static stability during isometric pushing. *Hum Factors*. 2005;47:536-549.

Gross KD, Hillstrom HJ. Noninvasive devices targeting the mechanics of osteoarthritis. *Rheum Dis Clin North Am*. 2008;34:755-776.

Halder AM, Zhao KD, Odriscoll SW, Morrey BF, An KN. Dynamic contributions to superior shoulder stability. *J Orthop Res*. 2001;19:206-212.

Helseth J, Hortobagyi T, Devita P. How do low horizontal forces produce disproportionately high torques in human locomotion? *J Biomech*. 2008;41:1747-1753.

Hodges PW, Cresswell AG, Daggfeldt K, Thorstensson A. In vivo measurement of the effect of intra-abdominal pressure on the human spine. *J Biomech*. 2001;34:347-353.

Hughes RE, An KN. Force analysis of rotator cuff muscles. *Clin Orthop Relat Res*. 1996:75-83.

Jorgensen MJ, Marras WS, Granata KP, Wiand JW. MRI-derived moment-arms of the female and male spine loading muscles. *Clin Biomech (Bristol, Avon)*. 2001;16:182-193.

Jorgensen MJ, Marras WS, Smith FW, Pope MH. Sagittal plane moment arms of the female lumbar region rectus abdominis in an upright neutral torso posture. *Clin Biomech (Bristol, Avon)*. 2005;20:242-246.

Kettler A, Hartwig E, Schultheiss M, Claes L, Wilke HJ. Mechanically simulated muscle forces strongly stabilize intact and injured upper cervical spine specimens. *J Biomech.* 2002;35:339-346.

Krevolin JL, Pandy MG, Pearce JC. Moment arm of the patellar tendon in the human knee. *J Biomech.* 2004;37:785-788.

Kuechle DK, Newman SR, Itoi E, Morrey BF, An KN. Shoulder muscle moment arms during horizontal flexion and elevation. *J Shoulder Elbow Surg.* 1997;6:429-439.

Kuechle DK, Newman SR, Itoi E, Niebur GL, Morrey BF, An KN. The relevance of the moment arm of shoulder muscles with respect to axial rotation of the glenohumeral joint in four positions. *Clin Biomech (Bristol, Avon).* 2000;15:322-329.

Labriola JE, Lee TQ, Debski RE, McMahon PJ. Stability and instability of the glenohumeral joint: the role of shoulder muscles. *J Shoulder Elbow Surg.* 2005;14:32S-38S.

Langenderfer JE, Patthanacharoenphon C, Carpenter JE, Hughes RE. Variability in isometric force and moment generating capacity of glenohumeral external rotator muscles. *Clin Biomech (Bristol, Avon).* 2006;21:701-709.

Langenderfer JE, Patthanacharoenphon C, Carpenter JE, Hughes RE. Variation in external rotation moment arms among subregions of supraspinatus, infraspinatus, and teres minor muscles. *J Orthop Res.* 2006;24:1737-1744.

Lee H, Granata KP, Madigan ML. Effects of trunk exertion force and direction on postural control of the trunk during unstable sitting. *Clin Biomech (Bristol, Avon).* 2008;23:505-509.

Lee SS, Piazza SJ. Inversion-eversion moment arms of gastrocnemius and tibialis anterior measured in vivo. *J Biomech.* 2008;41:3366-3370.

Li G, Pierce JE, Herndon JH. A global optimization method for prediction of muscle forces of human musculoskeletal system. *J Biomech.* 2006;39:522-529.

Maganaris CN. Imaging-based estimates of moment arm length in intact human muscle-tendons. *Eur J Appl Physiol.* 2004;91: 130-139.

Maganaris CN. In vivo measurement-based estimations of the moment arm in the human tibialis anterior muscle-tendon unit. *J Biomech.* 2000;33:375-379.

Maganaris CN, Baltzopoulos V, Tsaopoulos D. Muscle fibre length-to-moment arm ratios in the human lower limb determined in vivo. *J Biomech.* 2006;39:1663-1668.

Marras WS, Jorgensen MJ, Granata KP, Wiand B. Female and male trunk geometry: size and prediction of the spine loading trunk muscles derived from MRI. *Clin Biomech (Bristol, Avon).* 2001;16:38-46.

Mesfar W, Shirazi-Adl A. Biomechanics of the knee joint in flexion under various quadriceps forces. *Knee.* 2005;12:424-434.

Neumann DA. Biomechanical analysis of selected principles of hip joint protection. *Arthritis Care Res.* 1989;2:146-155.

Neumann DA. An electromyographic study of the hip abductor muscles as subjects with a hip prosthesis walked with different methods of using a cane and carrying a load. *Phys Ther.* 1999;79:1163-1173; discussion 1174-1176.

Neumann DA. Hip abductor muscle activity as subjects with hip prostheses walk with different methods of using a cane. *Phys Ther.* 1998;78:490-501.

Neumann DA. Hip abductor muscle activity in persons with a hip prosthesis while carrying loads in one hand. *Phys Ther.* 1996;76:1320-1330.

Neumann DA. Joint deformity and dysfunction: a basic review of underlying mechanisms. *Arthritis Care Res.* 1999;12:139-151.

Neumann DA, Cook TM. Effect of load and carrying position on the electromyographic activity of the gluteus medius muscle during walking. *Phys Ther.* 1985;65:305-311.

Neumann DA, Cook TM, Sholty RL, Sobush DC. An electromyographic analysis of hip abductor muscle activity when subjects are carrying loads in one or both hands. *Phys Ther.* 1992;72:207-217.

Neumann DA, Hase AD. An electromyographic analysis of the hip abductors during load carriage: implications for hip joint protection. *J Orthop Sports Phys Ther.* 1994;19:296-304.

Niu X, Latash ML, Zatsiorsky VM. Effects of grasping force magnitude on the coordination of digit forces in multi-finger prehension. *Exp Brain Res.* 2009;194:115-129.

Nozaki D. Torque interaction among adjacent joints due to the action of biarticular muscles. *Med Sci Sports Exerc.* 2009;41:205-209.

Ostermeier S, Friesecke C, Fricke S, Hurschler C, Stukenborg-Colsman C. Quadriceps force during knee extension after non-hinged and hinged TKA: an in vitro study. *Acta Orthop.* 2008;79:34-38.

Pandy MG. Moment arm of a muscle force. *Exerc Sport Sci Rev.* 1999;27:79-118.

Raison M, Gaudez C, Le Bozec S, Willems PY. Determination of joint efforts in the human body during maximum ramp pushing efforts. *J Biomech.* 2007;40:627-633.

Richards J, Thewlis D, Selfe J, Cunningham A, Hayes C. A biomechanical investigation of a single-limb squat: implications for lower extremity rehabilitation exercise. *J Athl Train.* 2008;43:477-482.

Riemer R, Hsiao-Wecksler ET. Improving net joint torque calculations through a two-step optimization method for estimating body segment parameters. *J Biomech Eng.* 2009;131:011007.

Robert T, Cheze L, Dumas R, Verriest JP. Validation of net joint loads calculated by inverse dynamics in case of complex movements: application to balance recovery movements. *J Biomech.* 2007;40:2450-2456.

Robertson DD, Debski RE, Almusa E, Armfield DR, Stone DA, Walker PS. Knee joint biomechanics: relevance to imaging. *Semin Musculoskelet Radiol.* 2003;7:43-58.

Rohlmann A, Bauer L, Zander T, Bergmann G, Wilke HJ. Determination of trunk muscle forces for flexion and extension by using a validated finite element model of the lumbar spine and measured in vivo data. *J Biomech.* 2006;39:981-989.

Ruckstuhl H, Krzycki J, Petrou N, et al. Shoulder abduction moment arms in three clinically important positions. *J Shoulder Elbow Surg.* 2009;18:632-638.

Schweizer A, Moor BK, Nagy L, Snedecker JG. Static and dynamic human flexor tendon-pulley interaction. *J Biomech.* 2009;42:1856-1861.

Smutz WP, Kongsayreepong A, Hughes RE, Niebur G, Cooney WP, An KN. Mechanical advantage of the thumb muscles. *J Biomech.* 1998;31:565-570.

Specogna AV, Birmingham TB, Hunt MA, et al. Radiographic measures of knee alignment in patients with varus gonarthrosis: effect of weightbearing status and associations with dynamic joint load. *Am J Sports Med.* 2007;35:65-70.

Thewlis D, Richards J, Bower J. Discrepancies in knee joint moments using common anatomical frames defined by different palpable landmarks. *J Appl Biomech.* 2008;24:185-190.

Tsaopoulos DE, Baltzopoulos V, Maganaris CN. Human patellar tendon moment arm length: measurement considerations and clinical implications for joint loading assessment. *Clin Biomech (Bristol, Avon).* 2006;21:657-667.

Tsaopoulos DE, Baltzopoulos V, Richards PJ, Maganaris CN. A comparison of different two-dimensional approaches for the determination of the patellar tendon moment arm length. *Eur J Appl Physiol.* 2009;105:809-814.

Tsaopoulos DE, Baltzopoulos V, Richards PJ, Maganaris CN. In vivo changes in the human patellar tendon moment arm length with different modes and intensities of muscle contraction. *J Biomech.* 2007;40:3325-3332.

Tsaopoulos DE, Maganaris CN, Baltzopoulos V. Can the patellar tendon moment arm be predicted from anthropometric measurements? *J Biomech.* 2007;40:645-651.

Walmsley RP, Pearson N, Stymiest P. Eccentric wrist extensor contractions and the force velocity relationship in muscle. *J Orthop Sports Phys Ther.* 1986;8(6):288-293.

Yanagawa T, Goodwin CJ, Shelburne KB, Giphart JE, Torry MR, Pandy MG. Contributions of the individual muscles of the shoulder to glenohumeral joint stability during abduction. *J Biomech Eng.* 2008;130:021024.

Zander T, Rohlmann A, Calisse J, Bergmann G. Estimation of muscle forces in the lumbar spine during upper-body inclination. *Clin Biomech (Bristol, Avon).* 2001;16 Suppl 1:S73-S80.

chapter 5

Friction

Introduction

Friction is a contact force that has a major effect on motion. Walking requires adequate friction between the sole of the foot and the floor. Friction is needed at initial contact and push-off, so that the foot will not slip forward or backward. On icy or other slick surfaces, one must bring the foot down perpendicular to the surface or a fall could result. Ramps must be built at low angles to reduce the friction problem. Wheelchairs may not be able to ascend a slippery slope. Crutches and canes are stable as a result of friction between their tips and the floor. Automobiles and other self-propelled vehicles rely on friction to start and stop and to go around curves.

Friction is used in many exercise devices to grade resistance to movement, as with a shoulder wheel, powder board, or stationary bicycle. Resistance is provided by friction for weight sleds for pushing and pulling and for cervical traction when a patient is supine. Gripping an object and opening jars require friction.

An important aspect in decubitus ulcers is the shear strain (friction) causing tears to cell walls and capillaries. Friction occurring within the body results in iliotibial band syndrome, bursitis, and tendonitis. A major concern of hand surgeons is the friction involved following tendon repair. Abrasions and blisters are the result of friction.

Prosthetic devices depend upon friction to control extension of the knee during gait and between surfaces in joint replacements. Friction may be a problem inside a prosthetic socket or between a cable and its housing.

Definitions

Friction is a force that opposes the relative motion between 2 objects that are in contact. It is a contact force that has a major effect on motion because it resists sliding of one object past another. However, it is a passive force that only appears when another force acts on the object.

LeVeau BF.
Biomechanics of Human Motion: Basics and Beyond for the Health Professions (pp 99-110).
© 2011 SLACK Incorporated

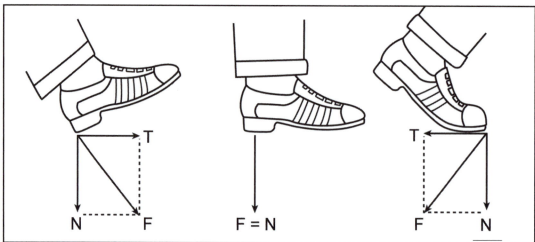

Figure 5-1. Force components on the foot during gait. Contact force (F), tangential or frictional force (T), and normal force (N).

The direction of the frictional force is dependent upon the direction in which the object tends to move. The frictional force always opposes the motion or potential motion of the object.

Probably the most common example of friction in everyday life is locomotion. We are able to walk and run because of friction between the ground and the foot (Figure 5-1). Try walking on ice or a very slick floor to illustrate this point. The coefficient of friction between the walking surface and crutch tips determine the angle with which the crutches can safely contact the ground. Wheelchairs need friction between the wheels and floor for starting and stopping. Some exercise devices such as the shoulder wheel (Figure 5-2), powder board (Figure 5-3), stationary bicycle (Figure 5-4), and pedal exerciser (Figure 5-5) use friction as resistance.

Friction also exists within the human body. Normally, ample lubrication is present as tendons slide within sheaths at sites of wear and articulating surfaces of joints are bathed in synovial fluid. Surfaces within a joint, however, may suffer wear damage as a result of friction. The type of materials used in total joint replacements has an effect on the wear caused by friction. Friction between the tendon and sheath affects the risk of tendon rupture and influences the tendon injury and repair. As one ages, the friction in joints (Figure 5-6) and tendon sheaths increases (Figure 5-7). Friction is an important component in the production of decubitus ulcers. Friction forces produce shear stress between the skin and underlying tissues. The resulting shear strain stretches and tears tissues, such as cell walls and capillaries. People who are ill, elderly, or paralyzed have greater tendency to suffer from the effects of friction on their tissues. Abrasions and blisters caused by friction are common occurrences seen daily by orthotists, prosthetists, physical therapists, athletic trainers, and other caregivers. Another example is friction between the prosthetic cable and the housing system that increases the amount of force needed to maneuver the prosthetic component.

The force of friction depends upon the normal force (N) between the 2 objects and the type of surface (μ) of each object. It does not depend upon the area between the 2 surfaces. The normal force is the force perpendicular to the surface (Figure 5-8). The normal force relates to how tightly the 2 materials are pressed together. The coefficient of friction is used to describe the effect of different surfaces and the roughness of the contact surfaces. Different types of materials have different coefficients of friction (Table 5-1). The formula for determining the magnitude of the frictional force is

$$F = \mu N$$

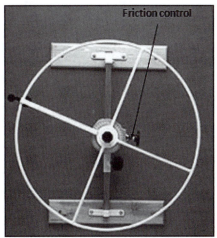

Figure 5-2. A shoulder wheel uses friction to offer resistance. Reprinted with permission from Patterson Medical/Sammons Preston, Bolingbrook, IL.

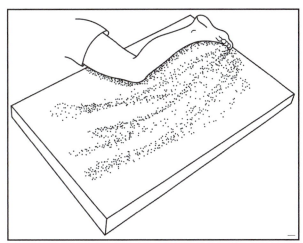

Figure 5-3. A powderboard uses powder to reduce friction resistance for exercise.

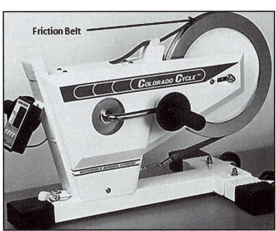

Figure 5-4. Stationary bicycles may use friction to provide resistance. Reprinted with permission from Patterson Medical/Sammons Preston, Bolingbrook, IL.

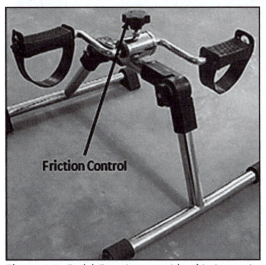

Figure 5-5. Pedal Exerciser provides friction resistance. Reprinted with permission from Patterson Medical/Sammons Preston, Bolingbrook, IL.

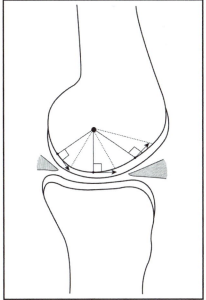

Figure 5-6. Friction occurs within a joint (see Figure 1-11).

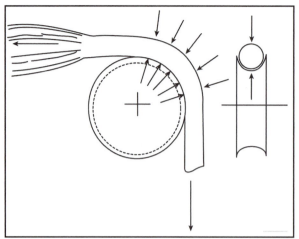

Figure 5-7. Friction on a tendon passing over a bone.

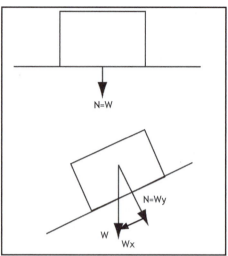

Figure 5-8. Friction along a level surface or an inclined plane. The normal (N, or W_y) force is perpendicular to the supporting surface.

TABLE 5-1

Coefficients of Friction (μ)

Surfaces	μ
Wood on wood, dry	0.23-0.50
Metal on metal, dry	0.15-0.20
Metal on tile	0.10-0.15
Metal on metal, greased	0.03-0.05
Rubber on concrete, dry	0.60-0.70
Rubber crutch tip on clean tile	0.30-0.40
Hard rubber cane tip on clean tile	0.18-0.22
Rubber crutch tip on rough wood	0.70-0.75
Hard rubber cane tip on rough wood	0.38-0.44

When motion occurs between the object and the supporting surface, μ decreases slightly to a lower value (dynamic friction). More force is needed to start an object moving than to keep it moving. Here, we will deal only with the friction that resists the start of motion (static friction) and not the friction as the object is moving.

Horizontal Plane

Suppose we wish to slide a large box across a room (Figure 5-9). We know the box and its contents weigh 100 lb. The coefficient of friction (μ) between the box and the floor is 0.30. By using the equation $F_f = \mu N$, we find that

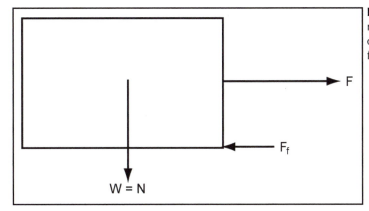

Figure 5-9. Sliding a box across a room: Applied force (F), weight (W) of box or normal force (N = W), and force of friction (F_f).

$$F_f = \mu N$$
$$F_f = 0.30 \times 100$$
$$F_f = 30 \text{ lb}$$

The force (F) needed to start sliding the box would be 30 lb.

How could we determine the coefficient of friction between the box and its supporting surface? We must know the weight of the box to be moved and have a device to measure the force to move the object. If the object weighed 100 lb (N) and the force (F_f) to begin moving the object was 30 lb, we can rearrange the equation:

$$F_f = \mu N$$
$$\frac{F_f}{N} = \mu$$
$$\frac{30 \text{ lb}}{100 \text{ lb}} = \mu$$
$$\mu = 0.30$$

When sliding a box, we must be concerned with 2 factors. We should always push horizontally. If the pushing force (F) has a component directed upward, part of the weight is being lifted and not directed toward sliding. If the pushing force (F) is directed downward, the downward component adds to the normal force and increases the need for a greater pushing force.

The second concern is the location of the application of the force to overcome friction (F_f). If this force is applied high on the box, the box may tip over instead of sliding. The following example illustrates this effect. Suppose we wish to slide a box with an evenly distributed load that is 6 ft tall and has a base of 3 ft by 3 ft (Figure 5-10). The center of mass of the box will be 3 ft high and 1.5 ft from the edge of the box. Where should the force be applied to slide the box and not to tip the box over? In this situation, we must use the second condition of equilibrium ($\Sigma M = 0$) as well as the friction formula ($F_f = \mu N$). The counterclockwise moment (CCW) is the weight of the box (100 lb) times the distance from the front edge of the box to the line of gravity (1.5 ft). The clockwise moment (CW) is the pushing force (F) times the distance the point of application is above the supporting surface (d_f). In a previous example, we found the force (F_f) to be 30 lb; the CW will be 30 lb times d_f. Solving for this equation (100 lb x 1.5 ft) + (30 lb x df) = 0, we find that d_f will equal 5 ft. If the point of application of the force is at or above 5 ft, the box will tip. If the force is applied below 5 ft, the box will slide. The mathematical solution is presented as follows:

Figure 5-10. Force to slide or tip a box. Applied force (F), weight (W) of box, and force of friction (F_f).

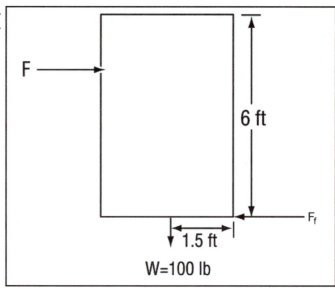

$$F_f = \mu N$$
$$\Sigma M = 0$$
$$\Sigma CCW + \Sigma CW = 0$$
$$(W \times d_{cg}) + (\text{-})(F_f \times d_f) = 0$$
$$(W \times d_{cg}) + (\text{-})(\mu N \times d_f) = 0$$
$$(100 \text{ lb} \times 1.5 \text{ ft}) + (\text{-})(0.30 \times 100 \text{ lb} \times d_f) = 0$$
$$(100 \text{ lb} \times 1.5 \text{ ft}) - (30 \text{ lb} \times d_f) = 0$$
$$(150 \text{ ft} \bullet \text{lb}) - (30 \text{ } d_f) = 0$$
$$150 \text{ ft} \bullet \text{lb} = 30 \text{ } d_f$$
$$\frac{150 \text{ ft} \bullet \text{lb}}{30 \text{ lb}} = d_f$$
$$d_f = 5 \text{ ft}$$

If the box had wheels, the coefficient of friction between the wheels and axles would set the value for μ in the friction formula.

Inclined Plane

Suppose that we must slide the box up an inclined plane or ramp (Figure 5-11). How much force would be needed to slide the box if the angle of the incline was 30 degrees? In this situation, the first condition of equilibrium ($\Sigma F = 0$) is used along with the resolution of forces and the friction equation. For the resolution of forces, the x-axis is set parallel to the surface of the inclined plane, and the y-axis is perpendicular to the ramp surface. The force (F) must overcome both the friction force (F_f) and the force component of the box weight (W_x), which is parallel to the surface of the ramp. The force of friction is determined by $F_f = \mu N$, where N equals the force component of the weight of the box (W_y), which is perpendicular to the ramp surface. The mathematical solution is as follows.

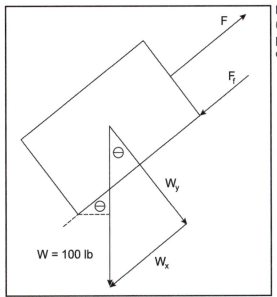

Figure 5-11. Sliding a box up a ramp. Applied force (F), weight (W) of box, normal force (N), weight component parallel to the supporting surface (W_x), angle of ramp (θ), and force of friction (F_f).

$$\Sigma F = 0$$
$$F + F_f + W_x = 0$$
$$\frac{W_x}{W} = \sin 30 \text{ degrees}$$
$$W_x = W \sin 30 \text{ degrees}$$
$$W_x = 100 \text{ lb} \times 0.5 = 50 \text{ lb}$$
$$\frac{W_y}{W} = \cos 30 \text{ degrees}$$
$$W_y = W \cos 30 \text{ degrees}$$
$$W_y = 100 \text{ lb} \times 0.866 = 86.6 \text{ lb}$$
$$F_f = \mu N = \mu W_y$$
$$F_f = 0.3 \times 86.6 \text{ lb} = 26 \text{ lb}$$
$$F + (\text{-})26 \text{ lb} + (\text{-})50 \text{ lb} = 0$$
$$F = 26 \text{ lb} + 50 \text{ lb}$$
$$F = 76 \text{ lb}$$

The general formula for this situation would be $F + (\mu W \cos\Theta) + (W \sin\Theta) = 0$.

If the force (F) were removed, what would happen to the box? Would it stay or slide down? To solve this problem, we use the previous general formula and set F equal to zero. Thus,

$$(\mu W \cos\Theta) + (W \sin\Theta) = 0;$$
$$\mu W \cos\Theta = 26 \text{ lb; and } W \sin\Theta = 50 \text{ lb}$$

Because $W \sin\Theta$ or Wx is greater than $(\mu W \cos\Theta)$ or F_f, then the box would slide back down the ramp.

Figure 5-12. With applied force removed, will the box slide down the ramp? Weight (W) of box, normal force (N), weight component parallel to the supporting surface (W_x), angle of ramp (θ), and force of friction (F_f).

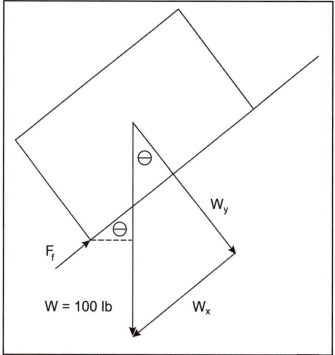

At what ramp angle would the box not slide down the ramp? Again, use the general formula, and set F equal to zero (Figure 5-12).

$$F + (\mu\ W\ \cos\Theta) + (W\ \sin\Theta) = 0$$

$$0 + (\mu\ W\ \cos\Theta) + (W\ \sin\Theta) = 0$$

$$\mu\ W\ \cos\Theta = W\ \sin\Theta$$

$$\mu = \frac{W\ \sin\Theta}{W\ \cos\Theta}$$

$$\mu = \frac{\sin\Theta}{\cos\Theta}, \text{ or } \frac{W_x}{W_y}$$

$$\mu = \tan\Theta$$

$$0.3 = \tan\Theta$$

$$\Theta = 16.7 \text{ degrees}$$

Another method to determine the coefficient of friction is to use the formula in the previous problem ($\mu = \tan\Theta$). If the supporting surface can be tilted, the angle of the surface can be changed until the object begins to slide. The coefficient of friction between the 2 surfaces is found to equal the tangent of that angle. If the object begins to slide at 30 degrees, then the coefficient of friction between the 2 surfaces would be $\mu = \tan 30$ degrees $= 0.577$.

Examples of the effect of friction on ramps include automobiles and trains going up slopes, walking up ramps and hills, and wheelchairs and crutches on ramps and hills. The slope and coefficient of friction can affect all of these situations.

Activities

1. Define friction and normal force.

2. Upon what factors does the force of friction depend?

3. Provide and discuss examples of frictional forces in the body, in clinical use, and in everyday activities.

4. What is the coefficient of friction between a 50-lb box and a carpeted floor if a force of 30 lb is needed to begin to slide the box?

5. A 150-lb patient is resting on a tilt table ($\mu = 0.45$). At what angle will the patient begin to slide?

6. If the coefficient of friction between a 70-lb box and a tile floor is 0.35, what force is necessary to slide the box? What would happen if the floor were polished and the coefficient of friction was reduced to 0.25? If the coefficient of friction between a therapist's shoes and the polished floor were 0.14, would the therapist be able to move the box?

7. What force would be necessary to pull a 70-lb box up a 20-degree ramp if the coefficient friction were 0.35? If the pulling force were removed, what would happen to the box?

8. An outside wooden ramp was built onto a person's home. The slope of the ramp is 15 degrees. Could a person in a wheelchair roll up the ramp if the coefficient were 0.45 between the wheels and the ramp? What would happen following a rain and the coefficient of friction were reduced to 0.25?

9. Find the required specifications for the slope of a ramp in a public building.

10. What effect does the angle of crutch tips have with the floor as a person ambulates with a swing-through gait? What effect would greater ambulation speed have on this situation?

11. A worker attempts to slide a 5-ft tall, 70-lb box along a concrete floor ($\mu = 0.55$). The base of the box is 4 ft by 4 ft with the mass evenly distributed in the box. How much force is needed to slide the box? What will happen if he pushes horizontally at the top of the box? Where on the box must he push to slide the box?

12. How much quadriceps muscle force is needed to extend the flexed leg on a powder board with 50 lb of cuff weights at the ankle? The perpendicular distance from the center of the knee joint to the patellar tendon is 2 in. The weight of the leg and foot is 10 lb with the combined center of mass located 10 in from the knee joint. The cuff weight resistance is 20 in from the knee joint. The coefficient of friction is 0.3 for the cuff weights and 0.4 for the leg. This muscle force will be able to lift how many pounds of cuff weights if the patient is sitting and extends the leg?

Answers

4. 0.6

5. 24.2 degrees

6. 24.5 lb; 17.5 lb; Yes, if the therapist weighs more than 125 lb.

7. 46.9 lb; It would slide down the ramp. 23.9 lb > 23.0 lb

8. Yes. After the rain, it could not go up.

11. >38.5 lb; tip over; lower than 3.63 ft

12. 170 lb; 12 lb

Suggested Reading

Amadio PC. Friction of the gliding surface. Implications for tendon surgery and rehabilitation. *J Hand Ther.* 2005;18:112-119.

Burnfield JM, Powers CM. Prediction of slips: an evaluation of utilized coefficient of friction and available slip resistance. *Ergonomics.* 2006;49:982-995.

Burnfield JM, Powers CM. The role of center of mass kinematics in predicting peak utilized coefficient of friction during walking. *J Forensic Sci.* 2007;52:1328-1333.

Burnfield JM, Tsai YJ, Powers CM. Comparison of utilized coefficient of friction during different walking tasks in persons with and without a disability. *Gait Posture.* 2005;22:82-88.

Cham R, Redfern MS. Changes in gait when anticipating slippery floors. *Gait Posture.* 2002;15:159-171.

Chang WR, Chang CC, Matz S. Available friction of ladder shoes and slip potential for climbing on a straight ladder. *Ergonomics.* 2005;48:1169-1182.

Chang WR, Kim IJ, Manning DP, Bunterngchit Y. The role of surface roughness in the measurement of slipperiness. *Ergonomics.* 2001;44:1200-1216.

Chang WR, Li KW, Filiaggi A, Huang YH, Courtney TK. Friction variation in common working areas of fast-food restaurants in the USA. *Ergonomics.* 2008;51:1998-2012.

Coert JH, Uchiyama S, Amadio PC, Berglund LJ, An KN. Flexor tendon-pulley interaction after tendon repair. A biomechanical study. *J Hand Surg Br.* 1995;20:573-577.

Domire ZJ, Karabekmez FE, Duymaz A, Rutar TS, Amadio PC, Moran SL. The effect of triangular fibrocartilage complex injury on extensor carpi ulnaris function and friction. *Clin Biomech (Bristol, Avon).* 2009; 24(10):807-811. Epub 2009 Sep 4

Dowson D. Tribological principles in metal-on-metal hip joint design. *Proc Inst Mech Eng H.* 2006;220:161-171.

Dowson D, Jin ZM. Metal-on-metal hip joint tribology. *Proc Inst Mech Eng H.* 2006;220:107-118.

Ellis R, Hing W, Reid D. Iliotibial band friction syndrome—a systematic review. *Man Ther.* 2007;12:200-208.

Fredericson M, Weir A. Practical management of iliotibial band friction syndrome in runners. *Clin J Sport Med.* 2006;16:261-268.

Hallan G, Lie SA, Havelin LI. High wear rates and extensive osteolysis in 3 types of uncemented total hip arthroplasty: a review of the PCA, the Harris Galante and the Profile/Tri-Lock Plus arthroplasties with a minimum of 12 years median follow-up in 96 hips. *Acta Orthop.* 2006;77:575-584.

Hanson JP, Redfern MS, Mazumdar M. Predicting slips and falls considering required and available friction. *Ergonomics.* 1999;42:1619-1633.

James R, Kesturu G, Balian G, Chhabra AB. Tendon: biology, biomechanics, repair, growth factors, and evolving treatment options. *J Hand Surg Am.* 2008;33:102-112.

Katta J, Jin Z, Ingham E, Fisher J. Biotribology of articular cartilage—a review of the recent advances. *Med Eng Phys.* 2008;30:1349-1363.

Kutsumi K, Amadio PC, Zhao C, Zobitz ME, An KN. Gliding resistance of the flexor pollicis longus tendon after repair: does partial excision of the oblique pulley affect gliding resistance? *Plast Reconstr Surg.* 2006;118:1423-1428; discussion 1429-1430.

Kutsumi K, Amadio PC, Zhao C, Zobitz ME, An KN. Measurement of gliding resistance of the extensor pollicis longus and extensor digitorum communis II tendons within the extensor retinaculum. *J Hand Surg Am.* 2004;29:220-224.

Manning DP, Jones C. The effect of roughness, floor polish, water, oil and ice on underfoot friction: current safety footwear solings are less slip resistant than microcellular polyurethane. *Appl Ergon.* 2001;32:185-196.

McCann L, Ingham E, Jin Z, Fisher J. Influence of the meniscus on friction and degradation of cartilage in the natural knee joint. Osteoarthritis *Cartilage.* 2009;17:995-1000.

McCann L, Ingham E, Jin Z, Fisher J. An investigation of the effect of conformity of knee hemiarthroplasty designs on contact stress, friction and degeneration of articular cartilage: a tribological study. *J Biomech.* 2009;42:1326-1331.

Menant JC, Perry SD, Steele JR, Menz HB, Munro BJ, Lord SR. Effects of shoe characteristics on dynamic stability when walking on even and uneven surfaces in young and older people. *Arch Phys Med Rehabil.* 2008;89:1970-1976.

Menant JC, Steele JR, Menz HB, Munro BJ, Lord SR. Effects of walking surfaces and footwear on temporo-spatial gait parameters in young and older people. *Gait Posture.* 2009;29:392-397.

Menz HB, Lord SR. Footwear and postural stability in older people. *J Am Podiatr Med Assoc.* 1999;89:346-357.

Moor BK, Nagy L, Snedeker JG, Schweizer A. Friction between finger flexor tendons and the pulley system in the crimp grip position. *Clin Biomech (Bristol, Avon).* 2009;24:20-25.

Niu X, Latash ML, Zatsiorsky VM. Effects of grasping force magnitude on the coordination of digit forces in multi-finger prehension. *Exp Brain Res.* 2009;194:115-129.

Redfern MS, Cham R, Gielo-Perczak K, et al. Biomechanics of slips. *Ergonomics.* 2001;44:1138-1166.

Schweizer A, Frank O, Ochsner PE, Jacob HA. Friction between human finger flexor tendons and pulleys at high loads. *J Biomech.* 2003;36:63-71.

Silva JM, Zhao C, An KN, Zobitz ME, Amadio PC. Gliding resistance and strength of composite sutures in human flexor digitorum profundus tendon repair: an in vitro biomechanical study. *J Hand Surg Am.* 2009;34:87-92.

Sun J, Walters M, Svensson N, Lloyd D. The influence of surface slope on human gait characteristics: a study of urban pedestrians walking on an inclined surface. *Ergonomics.* 1996;39:677-692.

Sun YL, Yang C, Amadio PC, Zhao C, Zobitz ME, An KN. Reducing friction by chemically modifying the surface of extrasynovial tendon grafts. *J Orthop Res.* 2004;22:984-989.

Taguchi M, Zhao C, Zobitz ME, An KN, Amadio PC. Effect of finger ulnar deviation on gliding resistance of the flexor digitorum profundus tendon within the A1 and A2 pulley complex. *J Hand Surg Am.* 2006;31:113-117.

Tanaka T, Amadio PC, Zhao C, Zobitz ME, An KN. Gliding resistance versus work of flexion—two methods to assess flexor tendon repair. *J Orthop Res.* 2003;21:813-818.

Tsai YJ, Powers CM. Increased shoe sole hardness results in compensatory changes in the utilized coefficient of friction during walking. *Gait Posture.* 2009;30:303-306.

Tsai YJ, Powers CM. The influence of footwear sole hardness on slip initiation in young adults. *J Forensic Sci.* 2008;53:884-888.

Uchiyama S, Amadio PC, Ishikawa J, An KN. Boundary lubrication between the tendon and the pulley in the finger. *J Bone Joint Surg Am.* 1997;79:213-218.

Williams S, Jalali-Vahid D, Brockett C, et al. Effect of swing phase load on metal-on-metal hip lubrication, friction and wear. *J Biomech.* 2006;39:2274-2281.

Yang C, Amadio PC, Sun YL, Zhao C, Zobitz ME, An KN. Tendon surface modification by chemically modified HA coating after flexor digitorum profundus tendon repair. *J Biomed Mater Res B Appl Biomater.* 2004;68:15-20.

Zatsiorsky VM, Latash ML. Prehension synergies. *Exerc Sport Sci Rev.* 2004;32:75-80.

Zhao C, Amadio PC, Zobitz ME, An KN. Resection of the flexor digitorum superficialis reduces gliding resistance after zone II flexor digitorum profundus repair in vitro. *J Hand Surg Am.* 2002;27:316-321.

Zhao C, Amadio PC, Zobitz ME, Momose T, Couvreur P, An KN. Gliding resistance after repair of partially lacerated human flexor digitorum profundus tendon in vitro. *Clin Biomech (Bristol, Avon).* 2001;16:696-701.

chapter 6

Dynamics

Objectives

1. Define motion and terms related to the study of motion.
2. Differentiate between kinematics and kinetics.
3. Provide and discuss examples of the study of motion in the body, in clinical use, and in everyday activities.
4. Differentiate between centrifugal force and centripetal force.
5. Solve problems related to kinematics.
6. Provide and discuss examples of kinetic approaches to evaluate forces in the body, in clinical use, and in everyday activities.
7. Analyze the resistance to acceleration offered by mass and inertia.
8. Relate the concepts of impulse and momentum.
9. Relate the concepts of work and energy.
10. Solve problems related to kinetics.

Introduction

The study of dynamics is invaluable in the health sciences disciplines. Biomechanical investigations have played major roles in the analysis of gait patterns, development of prosthetics and orthotics, analysis of muscle function in a variety of skills, the effect of movement on the joints of the body, the analysis of lifting and other ergonomic activities, and the analysis of injuries. By observing the characteristics of forces and applying Newton's Laws of Motion, characteristics of motion may be closely estimated. The basic principles of dynamics, along with a few examples, will be presented in this chapter. Many problems dealing with dynamics, however, are beyond the scope of this book.

Motion is defined as the continuous change in position. To be able to analyze motion, we must use the subdivision of mechanics known as dynamics. Dynamics is the study of motion. Dynamics is further subdivided into the areas of kinematics and kinetics. Kinematics is the study of the characteristics of motion, while kinetics is the study of the forces that affect motion.

LeVeau BF.
Biomechanics of Human Motion: Basics and Beyond for the Health Professions (pp 111-136).
© 2011 SLACK Incorporated

Kinematics

Kinematics allows us to describe the motion characteristics of displacement, velocity, and acceleration. The analysis of gait, for example, is concerned with the change of position of the body's center of mass and the angular motion of the limbs.

Displacement

Displacement is considered the change in position of an object. When every point on the object travels in a straight line, the displacement is linear or translatory (s) (Figure 6-1A). The displacement is angular or rotatory (θ) if every point on the object makes concentric circles around an axis (Figure 6-1B). During locomotion, the body as a whole tends to move in a linear fashion. However, this linear motion is brought about by angular motion of the limbs. Displacement is a vector quantity because it has magnitude and direction. Also note that linear motion is designated by Arabic letters, while angular motion is designated by Greek letters (Table 6-1).

Velocity

A certain amount of time is needed to change the position of an object. The velocity (v or ω) of an object is determined by the magnitude of the change in displacement (Δs or $\Delta \theta$) divided by the amount of time (t) taken to obtain the change in displacement, or

linear $\qquad v = \frac{\Delta s}{t}$

angular $\qquad \alpha = \frac{\Delta \theta}{t}$

Acceleration

The velocity of an object often changes as it moves. This change in velocity is called acceleration (a or α). If the velocity increases, the acceleration is positive. If the velocity decreases, the acceleration is negative and is sometimes referred to as deceleration. A certain amount of time is necessary for the velocity to change. Therefore, acceleration is the change in velocity (Δv or $\Delta \omega$) divided by the amount of time taken to obtain the change in velocity (t), or

linear $\qquad a = \frac{\Delta v}{t}$

angular $\qquad \alpha = \frac{\Delta \omega}{t}$

Linear/Angular Conversion

Note that the equations for angular motion are analogous to the equations for linear motion (see Table 6-1). Instead of being measured in terms of distance, angular motion is measure in terms of degrees or radians. The radian measurement can be used to relate the angular displacement to the linear displacement of a point on a rotating object. We could determine the linear displacement of the foot as it travels through angular motion. A radian (θ) is defined as the ratio of an arc (s) to the radius (r) of a circle (Figure 6-2A), or

$$\theta \text{ in radians} = \frac{s}{r}$$

The units of the arc and the radius are both linear and cancel each other. Therefore, the radian measure is considered unitless. When the length of the arc equals the distance from the axis to the moving point (the radius), the angle formed equals 57.3 degrees. Figure 6-2B shows that for $\frac{s}{r} = 1$, then $\theta = 57.3$ degrees. The relationship between linear and angular motion is

TABLE 6-1

Kinematic Characteristics

Characteristic	Linear	Angular
Displacement	s or d	θ
Velocity	$v = \Delta s/t$	$\omega = \Delta\theta/t$
Acceleration	$a = \Delta v/t$	$\alpha = \Delta\omega/t$

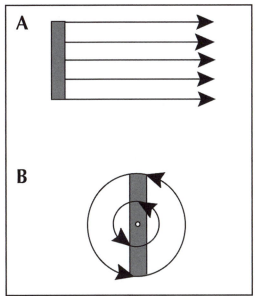

Figure 6-1. Types of displacement. (A) Linear. (B) Angular or rotatory.

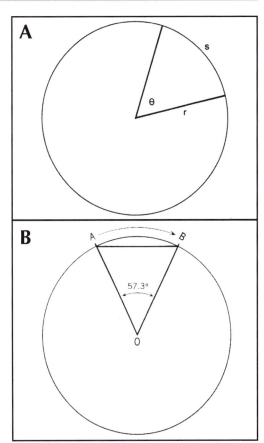

Figure 6-2. Relationship between linear and angular motion. Θ in radians = $\frac{s}{r}$, θ = angle, s = length of arc, and r = radius of object from axis.

related to the distance that the point of the object is from the axis of motion (r) as shown in the following equations:

$$s = r\theta$$
$$v = r\omega$$
$$a_t = r\alpha$$

Note that acceleration (a) is designated as a_t. As an object is rotated around an axis (Figure 6-3), 2 components of acceleration are involved. The object tends to fly away from the

Figure 6-3. Components of acceleration during angular motion. a = acceleration; a$_t$ = tangential acceleration; and a$_r$ = radial acceleration.

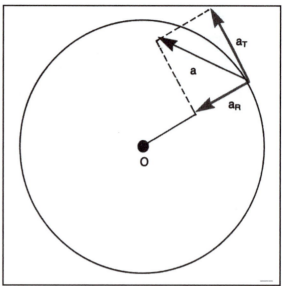

axis because of inertial force which, as in this situation, is also called centrifugal force. A force toward the axis (centripetal force) is needed to keep the object moving in the circular pattern and not moving further away from the axis. The a$_t$ notation (tangential acceleration) is the acceleration related to the inertial or centrifugal force. The notation of a$_r$ (radial acceleration) is the acceleration related to a constant change in direction caused by the centripetal force. In the case of the radial acceleration, the equation is

$$a_r = \frac{v^2}{r}$$

The entities of tangential acceleration (a$_t$) and radial acceleration (a$_r$) are components of the total acceleration (a) (see Figure 6-3). The total acceleration is determined by the equation

$$a^2 = a_t^2 + a_r^2$$

Example—Swinging Upper Limb

Suppose that an individual's upper limb is swinging back and forth (Figure 6-4). Assume for this problem that the elbow does not change its angular orientation. The elbow is located 11 in from the shoulder axis, and the hand is located 24 in from the shoulder axis. The angle for one swing of the upper limb is 65 degrees. Find the linear distance traveled by the elbow (E) and by the hand (H). The solution for this problem is as follows:

For the elbow:

$$1 \text{ radian} = 57.3 \text{ degrees}$$
$$\theta = \frac{65 \text{ degrees}}{57.3 \text{ degrees}}$$
$$\theta = 1.13 \text{ radians}$$
$$s = r\,\theta$$
$$s = 11 \text{ in} \times 1.13$$
$$s = 12.43 \text{ in}$$

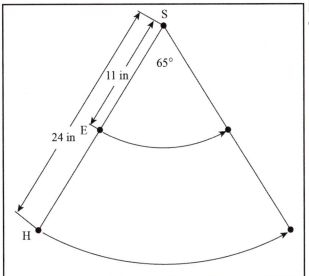

Figure 6-4. Upper limb swing. S is the shoulder, E is the elbow, and H is the hand.

For the hand:

$$1 \text{ radian} = 57.3 \text{ degrees}$$

$$\theta = \frac{65 \text{ degrees}}{57.3 \text{ degrees}}$$

$$\theta = 1.13 \text{ radians}$$

$$s = r\,\theta$$

$$s = 24 \text{ in} \times 1.13$$

$$s = 27.12 \text{ in}$$

Thus, the elbow moves 12.43 in and the hand moves 27.12 in.

Now, find the angular velocity of the limb and the linear velocities of the elbow and hand. The limb makes the excursion in 0.4 sec. The values of these characteristics are calculated as follows.

Angular velocity for the limb:

$$\theta = \frac{65 \text{ degrees}}{57.3 \text{ degrees}}$$

$$\theta = 1.13 \text{ radians}$$

$$\omega = \frac{\Delta\theta}{t}$$

$$\omega = \frac{1.13}{0.4 \text{ sec}}$$

$$\omega = \frac{2.82 \text{ radians}}{\text{sec}}$$

Linear velocity of the elbow:

$$v = r\omega$$

$$v = 11 \text{ in} \times 2.82 \text{ radians/sec}$$

$$v = 67.68 \text{ in/sec}$$

Linear velocity of the hand:

$$v = r\omega$$

$$v = 24 \text{ in} \times 2.82 \text{ radians/sec}$$

$$v = 31.08 \text{ in/sec}$$

Kinetics

As previously stated, kinetics is the study of the forces that affect motion. The forces presented in Chapter 1 can affect motion by initiating the motion of an object, by changing the direction of a moving object, or by stopping the motion of a moving object. By observing the characteristics of an object in motion and by applying Newton's Laws of motion, we may determine the magnitude of forces acting on an object.

In Chapter 1, we presented Newton's First Law of Motion that an object at rest tends to remain at rest and an object in motion tends to remain in motion at a constant velocity unless acted upon by an external force. In kinetics, we study the forces involved in changing the state of motion. Often, the forces acting on an object can be determined using Newton's Second Law of Motion, or what we can call the acceleration approach.

Force has been defined as a push or pull, but we can also define force as the attribute that tends to cause change in motion. The greater the force applied, the greater the potential for change in motion. As stated earlier, all objects have mass. Mass can be considered the amount of matter or the resistance to change in linear motion. Therefore, mass represents the amount of inertia of an object. More force is needed to change the motion of a large mass compared to that needed to change the motion of a small mass. These concepts establish the equation $a = \frac{F}{m}$, where acceleration (a) is an indication of the change in motion.

The rotatory equivalent of this concept is the equation, $\alpha = \frac{T}{I}$, where T is the torque or moment and I is the moment of inertia. The angular acceleration depends directly upon the torque applied (F x d) and inversely upon the moment of inertia ($I = \Sigma mr^2$), which was presented in Chapter 1.

Quite often, the characteristics of the motion can be determined by observation such as video, electrogoniometry, or other measuring devices. The process of forward or direct dynamics uses the force applied to the object to calculate its acceleration. On the other hand, the muscle and joint reaction forces are determined by evaluating the characteristics of motion and the effects of any external forces. In the process of inverse dynamics, acceleration of an object and any external forces such as ground reaction force (GRF) are used to determine the muscle force applied. See Figure 6-5 for models of direct and inverse dynamics.

ACCELERATION APPROACH

For statics in Chapter 4, we used the second condition of equilibrium to determine the muscle and joint forces to hold a load. For example, to hold the forearm horizontally without motion, the sum of the moments related to acceleration that act on the forearm and hand will equal zero. Therefore, the terms in the equation in the static situation include the moments caused by joint reaction, the muscles, gravity, and the load, or

$$\Sigma M = 0$$

$$\text{Joint} + \text{Muscle} + \text{Weight} + \text{Load} = 0$$

$$(J \times dj) + (M \times dm) + (W \times dw) + (L \times dl) = 0$$

When motion occurs, 2 other terms that resist change in motion are included in the equation. These are the moment of inertia of the forearm and hand ($I_w\alpha$) and the mass ($m_L a$) or moment of inertia ($I_L\alpha$) of the load. Because these moments resist the change in motion, they are in the opposite direction to the motion. If the load is attached to the body part such as with a cuff weight or dumbbell, load will move in an angular manner. If it is attached with a cord pulley system, the load will move linearly. Some types of resistance, such as a barbell, may provide

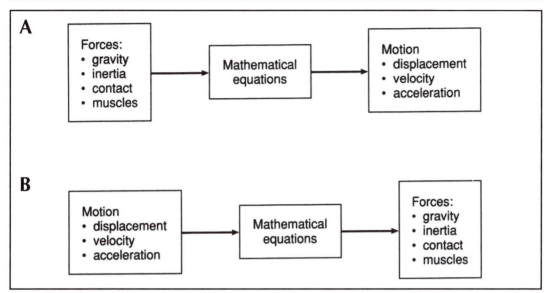

Figure 6-5. (A) Direct and (B) inverse dynamics study.

angular or linear resistance depending on what activity is being done. The following equations include the acceleration terms:

$$\Sigma M = \text{Joint} + \text{Muscle} + \text{Weight} + \text{Load} + \text{limb angular acceleration} + \text{load acceleration}$$

$$\Sigma M = (J \times dj) + (M \times dm) + (W \times dw) + (L \times dl) + I_w\alpha + (m_L \times a \times d_L, \text{ or } I_L\alpha)$$

In this equation, I_w is the moment of inertia of the body part, m_L is the mass of the load, a is the linear velocity of the load if the load moves linearly, I_L is the moment of inertia of the load if the load is moving in an arc with the limb, and α is the angular velocity of the limb. This equation is a simplified version of the second condition of equilibrium equation or Euler's equation. The sign for each term depends upon whether the moment is resisting the motion or assisting the motion. Remember that counterclockwise is considered positive and clockwise is considered negative.

Example—Fixed Pulley System

Suppose a client is using a single fixed pulley system to exercise the elbow flexor muscles (Figure 6-6). The client is sitting facing away from the wall. The arm is hanging down at the side with the upper limb in the anatomical position. Assume that the forearm and hand weigh 4 lb and its point of application at the center of mass is 6 in from the elbow joint. Appendix Table A-4 shows that the mass (m) of the forearm and hand is 0.1025 slugs, and Table A-5 shows the moment of inertia around the joint (I_0) is 6.26 slug • in^2. The load from the pulley system is 20 lb. The handle of the cord is held by the hand 13 in from the elbow joint. The cord at this beginning position is at a 90-degree angle with the forearm. As the client begins the exercise, the inertia of the forearm and hand and the load must be overcome. Because the limb and load are stationary, the initial velocity is zero. Therefore, during the early part of the movement, acceleration of the limb and load must occur. Let's determine the resistance to the limb movement caused by this acceleration during a slow movement and during a faster movement.

Figure 6-6. Patient moving a pulley weight.

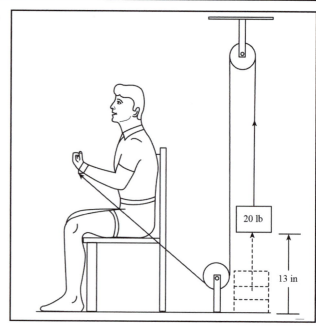

20 lb

13 in

Resistance of Load—Slow Movement

The acceleration during the first 0.4 sec of the elbow flexion movement of a slow movement is 4 ft/sec² (48 in/sec²). In this situation, 20 lb of force would be in the pulley cord if the load were being held stationary. What additional force (F) is developed in the pulley cord to accelerate the 20-lb weight (W)? The mass (m) of the 20-lb plate is determined by W = mg, where g equals the acceleration caused by gravity or 32.2 lb/sec². Thus,

$$W = F = ma$$

$$20 \text{ lb} = m \times 32.2 \text{ ft/sec}^2$$

$$\frac{20 \text{ lb}}{32.2 \text{ ft/sec}^2} = m$$

$$m = 0.62 \text{ slugs}$$

The mass of a 20-lb load is 0.62 slugs. The units of a slug are lb • sec²/ft. The linear resistance (or resisting force) of this load caused by the acceleration would be the mass of the load times the acceleration or F = ma. Therefore,

$$\text{Force} = \text{mass} \times \text{acceleration.}$$

$$0.62 \text{ slugs} \times 4 \text{ ft/sec}^2 = 2.48 \text{ lb}$$

The resistance caused by acceleration of this load would be this resisting force times the perpendicular distance that its point of attachment is to the elbow joint (m_L x a x d_L). The resistance for the load would be

$$\text{Force} \times \text{distance}$$

$$2.48 \text{ lb} \times 13 \text{ in} = 32.24$$

Therefore, the additional value for the resistance caused by the linear acceleration is 32.24 in • lb.

Resistance of Load—Faster Movement

The client wants to exercise at a faster rate of 15 ft/sec^2 (180 in/sec^2). In this case, the acceleration in the equation would change to 15 ft/sec^2. The linear resistance (or resisting force) of the faster moving load caused by the acceleration would be

$$\text{Force} = \text{mass x acceleration}$$
$$0.62 \text{ slugs x } 15 \text{ ft/sec}^2 = 9.3 \text{ lb}$$

The resistance for the faster load would be

$$\text{Force x distance}$$
$$9.3 \text{ lb x } 13 \text{ in} = 120.9 \text{ in} \bullet \text{lb}$$

Resistance of Limb During Movement

During this exercise, acceleration of the forearm also provides a resistance to the movement. In the slow exercise situation, the angular acceleration (α) was measured as 3.69 rad/sec^2, while in the faster movement, the angular acceleration was 13.85 rad/sec^2. The resistance to the acceleration of the limb is $I_w\alpha$.

Therefore, the resisting moment for limb acceleration is

slow movement   (6.26 slug $\bullet$ in^2 x 3.69 rad/sec^2) = 23.10 slug $\bullet$ in^2 rad/sec^2

faster movement   (6.26 slug $\bullet$ in^2 x 13.85 rad/sec^2) = 86.7 slug $\bullet$ in^2 rad/sec^2

Because the units of slugs is lb $\bullet$ sec^2/ft, the units must be made consistent in inches. Therefore, the term (1 ft/12 in) must be introduced to the angular acceleration component. The resistance in inch $\bullet$ pound would be

slow movement   (23.10 slug $\bullet$ in^2 rad/sec^2 x 1 ft/12 in) = 1.93 in $\bullet$ lb

faster movement   (86.7 slug $\bullet$ in^2 rad/sec^2 x 1 ft/12 in) = 7.23 in $\bullet$ lb

The resistance terms caused by acceleration (ma and Iα) would be added to the static situation of the limb.

Using Cuff Weight Instead of Pulley System

To determine the magnitude of resistance to forearm flexion if the load were a cuff weight or dumbbell instead of a plate in a pulley system, the term $I_L\alpha$ would be used. Remember that, for the moment of inertia, $I = \Sigma mr^2$. In the situation of the cuff weight, the radius (r) of the mass would be considered to be the distance of the load to the axis of the elbow or 13 in. The equation for the resistance to acceleration would be

$$I_L\alpha = mr^2\alpha$$

Thus, for the slow movement, the term would be

$$(0.62 \text{ slug x } 13 \text{ in x } 13 \text{ in x } 3.69 \text{ rad})$$

Therefore, the resistance to limb acceleration is

slow movement   (0.62 slug x 269 in^2 x 3.69 rad/sec^2) = 615.42 slug $\bullet$ in^2 rad/sec^2

faster movement   (0.62 slug x 269 in^2 x 13.85 rad/sec^2) = 2309.9 slug $\bullet$ in^2 rad/sec^2

Because the units of slugs is lb $\bullet$ sec^2/ft, the units must be made consistent in inches. Therefore, the term (1 ft/12 in) must be introduced to the angular acceleration component. The resistance in inch $\bullet$ pound would be

slow movement   (615.42 slug $\bullet$ in^2 rad/sec^2 x 1 ft/12 in) = 51.29 in $\bullet$ lb

faster movement   (2309.9 slug $\bullet$ in^2 rad/sec^2 x 1 ft/12 in) = 192.49 in $\bullet$ lb

One of the concepts that you must remember about movement such as elbow flexion is that positive acceleration occurs at the beginning of the movement, and negative acceleration occurs near the end of the movement. Constant velocity may exist between the positive and negative accelerations. The force used to accelerate a load does not occur throughout the movement.

Impulse-Momentum

Linear Motion

In some situations, force is applied over a time period, or collisions occur. An adaptation of the acceleration formula gives the impulse-momentum approach. The acceleration formula with linear motion is $a = \frac{F}{m}$, or more commonly known as $F = ma$. From the study of kinematics, we saw that acceleration is the change of velocity during a specific time period $(a = \frac{\Delta v}{t})$. The formula $F = ma$ becomes $F = \frac{m\Delta v}{t}$, the magnitude of force needed to change the velocity of an object in a given time. By multiplying both sides by t, this equation becomes $Ft = m\Delta v$, or $Ft = mv_2 - mv_1$. Force acting over a period of time (Ft) is called impulse, while a moving mass (mv) is called the momentum. The change in momentum is designated by $mv_2 - mv_1$, or $m\Delta v$. This change from $a = \frac{F}{m}$ to $Ft = mv_2 - mv_1$ is illustrated as follows.

$$a = \frac{F}{m}$$

$$F = ma$$

$$F = \frac{m\Delta v}{t}$$

$$Ft = m\Delta v$$

$$Ft = mv_2 - mv_1$$

A force applied over a period of time is a way to control the momentum of an object. The greater the magnitude of force, the less time is needed to change the momentum of an object. When someone runs into a wall, a large force is applied by the wall, and the stop is sudden. If a pilot ejects from a burning airplane and lands on a snow-covered mountain slope, his momentum (his mass times his falling velocity) may take a long time to become zero $(v = 0)$ as he slides down the mountain side. In this situation, the force (F) is less because the time (t) is large. Examples of impulse-momentum occur often in everyday life. This concept is involved any time a collision occurs, such as a car and a truck, a fist and a jaw, a running back and a linebacker, and a bat and a ball. In exercise, the concept is also important. When lifting weights, the weight begins with a velocity of zero. A force is applied to the weight, and its velocity is increased. The greater the force applied, the faster the weight will move. If a weight is moving at a high velocity, a large force is needed to stop it quickly. Less force is needed to stop the motion of an object if the time of force application can be lengthened. An example of this situation is the attempt to catch an object like a baseball, egg, or water balloon. If the hand is held rigid, less time for the catch occurs, and the catch will be unsuccessful. However, if the hand withdraws, allowing more time for the catch, chances for a successful catch are improved. The use of padding for helmets and covering hard surfaces also use the concept of impulse and momentum because the padding allows time for the motion to decrease in magnitude. Impulse and momentum are directly related to Newton's First Law (Law of Inertia).

The Law of Conservation of Momentum is related to Newton's Third Law of Motion (Law of Reaction). When 2 objects collide, the magnitude of force on one object is the same but in the opposite direction as the force on the second object. The time for the collision is the same for both objects. The impulse on each object is the same. Therefore, the change in momentum for both objects is the same, but in the opposite direction, or $m_2v_1 - m_1v_1 = -m_2v_2 - m_1v_2$. As a collision occurs, for example, one object will decrease its velocity as the other increases its velocity an equal amount.

Rotatory Motion

Impulse-momentum concept also occurs during rotatory motion. From the formula $T = I\alpha$, the relationship of $T = I\frac{\Delta\omega}{t}$ can be obtained. Further manipulation of the equation gives $Tt = I\Delta\omega$, where Tt is the angular impulse and $I\Delta\omega$ is the angular momentum. The change in angular momentum is $I\omega_2 - I\omega_1$. A torque applied over a period of time will change the angular momentum of a rotating object.

$$\alpha = \frac{T}{I}$$
$$T = I\alpha$$
$$T = I\frac{\Delta\omega}{t}$$
$$Tt = I\Delta\omega$$
$$Tt = I\omega_2 - I\omega_1$$

In angular movement of the human body, the moment of inertia ($I = \Sigma mr^2$) can be changed. Therefore, the change in momentum can be written as $mr_1^2\omega_1 - mr_2^2\omega_2$, where the mass is constant, but the distribution of the mass and the angular velocity change. As an individual is walking, the elbows are more extended, and the knees do not flex a great amount. However, as the individual begins to run, the elbows become more flexed (decrease r), and the knees flex more (decrease r) during the swing phase so that these limbs may move faster without a major increase in shoulder muscle force. The change in the distribution of mass makes the body more efficient by requiring less muscle force to accelerate and decelerate the limbs.

The concept of angular momentum is important in many athletic events, such as ice skating, gymnastics, and diving, as well as in locomotion. Often, as the athlete spins or rotates in the air, no outside force is applied to the body. Therefore, the impulse will equal zero. If $Ft = 0$, then $mr_1^2\omega_1 - mr_2^2\omega_2 = 0$, or $mr_1^2\omega_1 = mr_2^2\omega_2$. As an ice skater is spinning, if she brings her arms in closer to her axis of spin (decreasing r), she will spin faster. If she moves her hands away from her body (increasing r), her spin will decrease or stop. As a diver tucks, bringing the knees and arms toward the chest, the body rotates rapidly. A tighter tuck produces a faster rotation. Extending the arms and straightening the hips and knees causes the rotation of the body to slow down or cease.

Angular impulse and momentum are related to the cause of injuries. As the leg swings through during sprinting, the sprinter must rapidly decelerate the leg for foot contact on the ground. This change in velocity must take place in a very short period of time ($I\frac{\Delta\omega}{t}$). A great magnitude of torque by the hamstring muscles is necessary to cause this change of motion. Because the point of application of the hamstring muscles does not change, the force produced by the hamstring muscles must have a great magnitude. The hamstring muscles must be capable to produce this force in an eccentric fashion, or part of the muscle may rupture (hamstring strain). A similar situation occurs as a pitcher is throwing a baseball. The external rotator muscles of the humerus must contract rapidly with a great amount of force to decelerate the upper limb after the ball is released. The specialty area of prosthetics and orthotics involves impulse and momentum. A patient wearing an ankle-foot orthosis (AFO) has an added mass (m) at a distance from the knee joint (r). This additional mass increases the moment of inertia by mr^2. Heavy boots and ankle weights will have a similar effect on the leg. A prosthesis must have the appropriate mass and distribution of mass to be able to function similarly to the unamputated limb.

Work-Energy

Work and energy are closely related. When work is done on an object, a change in the energy of the object occurs (work-energy theorem). The work applied and the change in energy are equal and are measured in the same units. The work-energy approach to analyze movement depends upon the position or velocity of the body or object involved. Work involves a force or forces that cause an object to move a given distance or to change its velocity. The work can occur linearly, or it can be rotational. The distance moved is along the line of application and in the direction of the force performing the linear work. Positive work occurs while lifting an object (Figure 6-7), sliding an object against friction (Figure 6-8), or causing strain deformation (Figure 6-9). The term negative work is used when the object is lowered from a height or the force is used to control the return of the strain deformation to its original position. Muscles are considered to be doing positive work during concentric contractions and doing negative work during eccentric contractions. As stated in Chapter 1, the equation for linear work is

$$W = F \times s = mas$$

As a box is lifted from the floor onto a table, work (W) has been done by applying a force (F) and moving the box a distance (s) vertically against the force of gravity. The moving box has kinetic energy (KE) depending upon its mass (m) and its change in velocity squared $(v_f - v_o)^2$, or

$$KE = \tfrac{1}{2}m(v_f - v_o)^2$$

This equation shows that the magnitude of kinetic energy depends upon the change in the velocity of the object. The greater the velocity change, the greater the kinetic energy of the object is. An object may begin or end its motion at rest, such as the box placed on the table. In this situation, the final velocity (v_f) is zero. Thus, the common equation for kinetic energy is

$$KE = \tfrac{1}{2}mv^2$$

When the box is resting on the table, it has no kinetic energy, but it has gained potential energy. Chapter 1 presented that an object contains stored energy or potential energy (PE) because of its height above a reference point. The weight (W = mg) of the box and its height above the floor (h) provide the equation of potential energy of the box on the table with reference to the floor, or

$$PE = mgh$$

Note that the work done to lift the box from the floor (W = Fs) was equal to the force to lift the box against gravity (weight of the box, mg) times the distance lifted above the floor (s = h). Therefore,

$$W = Fs = mgh = PE$$

WORK AGAINST GRAVITATIONAL LOAD

The work done using elbow flexor muscles to lift a 20-lb pulley weight 16 in against the force of gravity (see Figure 6-6) can be calculated as follows:

$$W = F \times s = mas$$
$$W = 20 \text{ lb} \times 16 \text{ in}$$
$$W = 320 \text{ in} \cdot \text{lb, or } 26.67 \text{ ft} \cdot \text{lb}$$

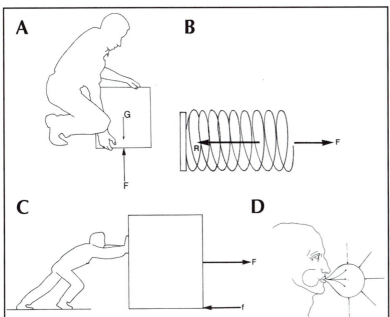

Figure 6-7. Examples of work. (A) Lifting against gravity. (B) Overcoming the force of a spring. (C) Pushing against friction. (D) Stretching an elastic balloon.

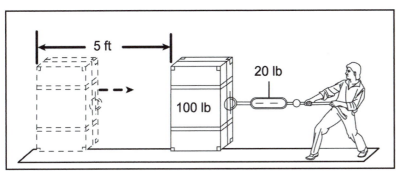

Figure 6-8. Work against friction.

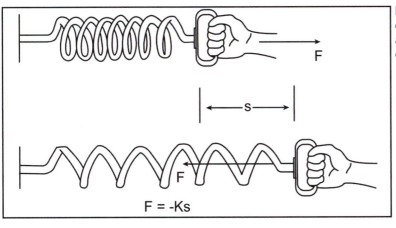

Figure 6-9. Work against elastic resistance. F is the applied force, and s is the distance moved.

$$F = -Ks$$

As work is applied to lift the 20-lb weight, potential energy (PE) is stored because of the gravitational force (mg) and its height (h) above the ground or other reference point. The potential energy gained is equal to the work done, or

$$W = PE = mgh$$

WORK CLIMBING STAIRS

Lifting objects is a common endeavor, but lifting one's own body is also common and requires work to be done (Figure 6-10). Climbing stairs is the most common way that one lifts the body. The work done in this situation depends on the weight of the individual's body, the height of each step, and the number of steps. If a 150-lb individual climbs 10 steps that are each 8-in high, how much work does the individual do to climb the stairs?

$$W = F \text{ x } s;$$
$$s = 8 \text{ in x } 10 \text{ steps} = 80 \text{ in}$$
$$W = 150 \text{ lb x } 80 \text{ in}$$
$$W = 12,000 \text{ in} \cdot \text{lb}$$
$$W = 12,000 \text{ in} \cdot \text{lb x } \left(\frac{1 \text{ ft}}{12 \text{ in}}\right)$$
$$W = 1,000 \text{ ft} \cdot \text{lb}$$

The 150-lb individual does 1,000 ft • lb of work to climb 10 8-in steps. You can use your weight and the height of stairs that you climb to determine the amount of work you do as you go up stairs. The work done while performing on a stepping exercise device can be determined using the same equation.

WORK AGAINST FRICTIONAL LOAD

When performing work against friction, the work (W) equals the force (F) needed to move the object times the distance (s) the object is moved. Therefore, work can be done when sliding a box along a surface. If a 50-lb box is pushed 20 ft along a level floor with a constant velocity, how much work would be done if the coefficient of sliding friction (μ) were 0.3? To solve this problem, the amount of force to slide the box and the distance the box moved are necessary.

$$F = \mu N$$
$$F = 0.3 \text{ x } 50 \text{ lb}$$
$$F = 15 \text{ lb}$$

Thus, the force to move the box is 15 lb. The box is moved 20 ft. Therefore, the work to move the box can be found by multiplying the force times the distance the box moved or

$$W = F \text{ x } s$$
$$W = 15 \text{ lb x } 20 \text{ ft}$$
$$W = 300 \text{ ft} \cdot \text{lb}$$

The work done to slide the box along the floor for 20 ft is 300 ft • lb. Note that the work in this case has not gained any potential energy. Why not? The kinetic energy during the sliding motion is converted to heat instead of mechanical energy.

Suppose we wish to slide the 50-lb box up a 20-degree ramp having a coefficient of friction of 0.3. How much work is done when the box reaches the surface of the loading dock 3 ft above the ground? If the loading dock is 3 ft above the ground and the angle of incline is 20 degrees, then the length of the incline (s) would be calculated to be

$$\frac{3 \text{ft}}{s} = \sin \theta$$
$$\frac{3 \text{ft}}{\sin \theta} = s$$
$$\sin \theta = 0.342$$
$$s = 8.77 \text{ ft}$$

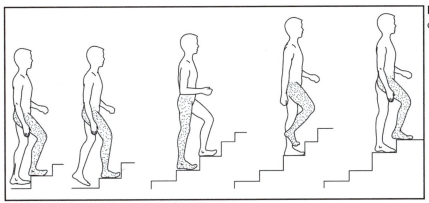

Figure 6-10. Work climbing stairs.

The work (W) done would be the force (F) to move the box times the distance (s) the box is moved. We know that the box would move the length of the ramp, but what is the force (F) to move the box? Referring to Chapter 5, we find that the force to slide a box up a ramp depends upon 1) the resistance caused by friction ($F_f = \mu N$ or $\mu\, W \cos \theta$), and 2) the weight component of the box parallel to the surface of the ramp (W_x or $W \sin \theta$).

$$\Sigma F = 0$$
$$F + F_f + W_x = 0$$
$$F + (\mu\, W \cos\theta) + (W \sin\theta) = 0$$
$$\frac{W_x}{W} = \sin 20 \text{ degrees}; \; W_x = W \sin 20 \text{ degrees}$$
$$W_x = 50 \text{ lb} \times 0.342 = 17.1 \text{ lb}$$
$$\frac{W_y}{W} = \cos 20 \text{ degrees}; \; W_y = W \cos 20 \text{ degrees}$$
$$W_y = 50 \text{ lb} \times 0.94 = 47 \text{ lb}$$
$$F_f = \mu N = \mu W_y$$
$$F_f = 0.3 \times 47 \text{ lb} = 14.1 \text{ lb}$$
$$F + (-)14.1 \text{ lb} + (-)17.1 \text{ lb} = 0$$
$$F = 14.1 \text{ lb} + 17.1 \text{ lb}$$
$$F = 31.2 \text{ lb}$$

The work done is as follows.

$$W = F \times s$$
$$W = 31.2 \text{ lb} \times 8.77 \text{ ft}$$
$$W = 273.6 \text{ ft} \cdot \text{lb}$$

Note that the work done to slide the box up the ramp (273.6 ft • lb) with a length of 8.77 ft is slightly less than to slide the box 20 ft along a level floor (300 ft • lb). How would this problem relate to a patient in a wheelchair going up a ramp?

WORK AGAINST ELASTIC LOAD

A force (F) is applied to deform or change the length (s) of an elastic material such as a spring or elastic band that has a given stiffness (k). This deformation requires work to be done as the force is applied over the length change. The force at any specific length of the material with a stiffness of k is

$$F = -ks$$

The minus sign indicates that the restoring force is opposite in direction of the applied force. The work done to deform the material over the entire length change is shown by the equation

$$W = \frac{1}{2}ks^2$$

Suppose a client is using an elastic band in the hand to exercise the elbow flexor muscles (Figure 6-11). At the beginning of the elbow flexion, the force (F_o) of the band is zero. As the band is lengthened, its resistance (restoring force) to the applied force increases in a linear fashion. The elbow flexion is ceased after the angle traversed 76 degrees and the band was lengthened 16 in. To keep this example simple, assume that the band maintains a 90-degree angle with the forearm throughout the range of motion. The restoring force (F_s) produced by the band in the lengthened position is 40 lb.

Therefore, the average restoring force (F_a) for the entire flexion motion is

$$F_a = \frac{(F_o + F_s)}{2}$$
$$F_a = \frac{(0 + F_s)}{2} = \frac{F_x}{2}$$
$$F_x = -ks$$
$$F_a = \frac{-ks}{2}$$

The stiffness of this elastic band (k) is 2.548 lb/in. To determine the work (W) accomplished on the band, the average force (F_a) must be used in the work equation. The work done in this situation is

$$W = F_a \times s$$
$$W = \frac{ks}{2} \times s, \text{ or } \frac{ks^2}{2}$$
$$W = \frac{[(2.548 \text{ lb/in}) \times (16 \text{ in})^2]}{2}$$
$$W = 326.1 \text{ in} \cdot \text{lb, or}$$
$$W = (326.1 \text{ in} \cdot \text{lb}) \times (\frac{1 \text{ ft}}{12 \text{ in}}) = 27.18 \text{ ft} \cdot \text{lb}$$

In this situation, each flexion repetition produces 27.18 ft • lb of work. Note that the minus was not used in this equation because the minus sign related to the direction of the restoring force, not to the direction of the applied force doing the work.

As work is applied to deform an elastic material, potential energy (PE) is stored within the material. The potential energy gained is equal to the work done, or

$$W = PE = \frac{1}{2}ks^2$$

WORK AGAINST DAMPING LOAD

As stated in Chapter 1, the magnitude for rotatory work is determined by using the torque applied to move a lever (T) times the magnitude of the angular displacement of the lever (Θ), or

$$W = T \times \Theta$$

The angular work equation must be used to determine the amount of work accomplished with an exercise device that employs a damping mechanism for resistance (for example: hydraulic, pneumatic, and friction).

Suppose a client is performing elbow flexion exercises on a hydraulic exercise device set to provide 20 lb of resistance (F) at the handpiece (Figure 6-12). The lever length is 13 in long (d) with the axis set adjacent to the elbow. During the exercise, the elbow is flexed 76 degrees for

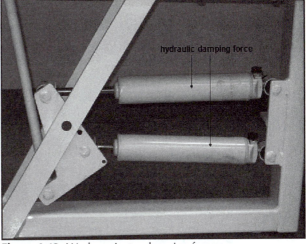

Figure 6-12. Work against a damping force.

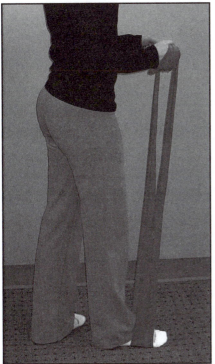

Figure 6-11. Work against an elastic load.

each repetition. How much work is done by the elbow flexor muscles with one repetition? How much work is done by the elbow flexor muscles with 10 repetitions?

$$W = T \times \theta$$
$$T = Fd = 20 \text{ lb} \times 13 \text{ in} = 260 \text{ in lb (torque)}$$
$$\theta = \frac{76 \text{ degrees}}{57.3 \text{ degrees}} = 1.33 \text{ radians}$$
$$W = 260 \text{ in} \cdot \text{lb} \times 1.33 \text{ radians}$$
$$W = 345.8 \text{ in} \cdot \text{lb (work) or}$$
$$W = 345.8 \text{ in} \cdot \text{lb} \times \frac{1 \text{ ft}}{12 \text{ in}}$$
$$W = 28.8 \text{ ft} \cdot \text{lb (work)}$$

In this situation, each flexion repetition produces 28.8 ft • lb of work. Ten repetitions of flexion would produce 288 ft • lb of work.

In this type of device, the hydraulic resistance may be set at 30 lb of resistance for elbow extension. Work done during one repetition of elbow extension would be

$$W = T \times \theta$$
$$T = Fd = 30 \text{ lb} \times 13 \text{ in} = 390 \text{ in lb (torque)}$$
$$\theta = \frac{76 \text{ degrees}}{57.3 \text{ degrees}} = 1.33 \text{ radians}$$
$$W = 390 \text{ in lb} \times 1.33 \text{ radians}$$
$$W = 518.7 \text{ in} \cdot \text{lb (work) or}$$
$$W = 518.7 \text{ in} \cdot \text{lb} \times \frac{1 \text{ ft}}{12 \text{ in}}$$
$$W = 43.2 \text{ ft} \cdot \text{lb (work)}$$

The elbow extensor muscles concentrically contract, producing 43.2 ft • lb of work.

The related energy as work is applied to a damping type of device is not stored as potential energy, but is dissipated as heat.

EXAMPLES OF ENERGY CHANGE

A simple example of change in mechanical energy is when an object is dropped from a height (Figure 6-13). For example, as a 50-lb box is being held 3 ft above the floor, its potential energy is mgh = (50 lb x 3 ft) = 150 ft • lb. Because it is not moving (v = 0), its kinetic energy is $\frac{1}{2}mv^2$ or 0. As the box falls with constant acceleration from the force of gravity, the kinetic energy increases, and as the box approaches the floor, its potential energy decreases (Figure 6-14). Just before the box strikes the floor, its potential energy is zero, and its kinetic energy is 150 ft • lb. No measurable energy is dissipated as heat or sound.

Some situations of exchange of energy include gravity and elastic force in concert. Once an individual begins jumping on a trampoline (Figure 6-15), gravity pulls the individual down, and elastic force pushes the individual into the air. At the highest point of the activity, the individual's potential energy because of gravity is maximum (PE = mgh). At the lowest point of the activity, the trampoline surface is stretched, and it has its maximum potential energy (for an elastic material, PE = $\frac{1}{2}$mks). The kinetic energy varies from zero to maximum to zero from the highest point to the lowest point and back. If the individual does not add force, the activity will soon cease because of the energy dissipated by the trampoline as heat and sound. Other objects that combine the force of gravity and elastic force are various types of balls, a vaulting pole, a pogo stick, and prosthetic feet.

Buoyant force can apply kinetic energy to an object or body as well (Figure 6-16). If an object that is less dense than water is forced down below its surface (F x d), when released, the object will rapidly ascend and shoot out above the water's surface. Buoyant force can be used as a mild resistance for muscle strengthening exercise.

A pneumatic device allows the air in a cylinder to be compressed by a moving piston followed by an increased pressure within the cylinder. As the pressure is increased, the motion of the piston is opposed. Potential energy is developed within the compressed gas. The piston is then pushed back in the other direction.

A common activity in which energy is constantly being exchanged is the various modes of ambulation. The center of mass of the body is continually being raised and falling. The faster the mode of ambulation, the more rapidly the energy is exchanged. Also, during ambulation, energy is stored and released in muscles and tendons for more economical locomotion. The body segments are continually transferring energy from one segment to the adjacent segments.

MECHANICAL ENERGY LOSS

Most activities will dissipate energy over a period of time. A dropped bouncing ball illustrates this concept. Some activities, however, dissipate the energy very rapidly. Friction force on exercise bicycles is designed to provide resistance without returning mechanical energy to the system. Eddy currents from electromagnetic force do the same in elliptical exercise devices. Damping effects in hydraulic devices dissipate the energy from the work applied. Protective devices made of energy-absorbing materials, such as foam in pads, helmets, and the SACH foot, reduce the chance of injury from application of large forces.

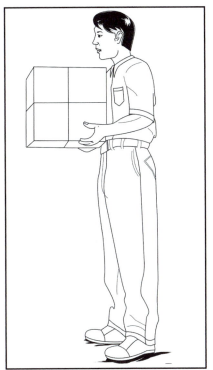

Figure 6-13. Potential energy while holding a box.

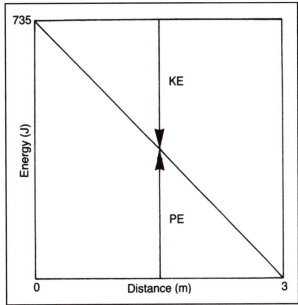

Figure 6-14. Graph of the relative values of potential and kinetic energy related to total energy.

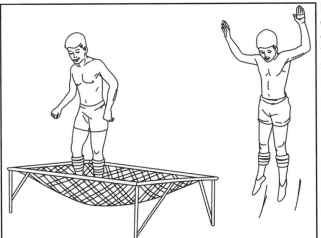

Figure 6-15. Jumping on a trampoline demonstrates change in potential and kinetic energy. Potential energy at the height of the jump and when the trampoline is fully stretched.

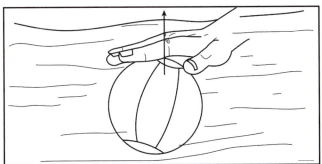

Figure 6-16. Energy related to a buoyant force. The potential energy is present as the ball is held under water. Kinetic energy occurs as the ball is released and it moves upward.

Power

Power, as defined in Chapter 1, is the rate of doing work ($P = \frac{W}{t}$), the rate of force acting at a specific velocity ($P = Fv$; $P = T\omega$), or the rate of expending energy

$$P = \tfrac{1}{2}m(v_f^2 - v_i^2); P = \tfrac{1}{2}I(\omega_f^2 - \omega_i^2)$$

Earlier in this chapter, you determined the amount of work for an individual to climb stairs. The stairs may be traversed slowly or rapidly to perform the same amount of work. However, the more time that is taken to climb the stairs, the less power is used. The work done by a 150-lb individual climbing 10 8-in steps was 1,000 ft • lb. If the individual climbs the stairs in 15 sec, the power output is

$$P = \frac{W}{t}$$
$$P = \frac{1{,}000 \text{ ft} \bullet \text{lb}}{15 \text{ sec}}$$
$$P = 66.67 \text{ ft} \bullet \text{lb/sec}$$

If the individual climbs the stairs in 5 sec, the power output will be

$$P = \frac{W}{t}$$
$$P = \frac{1{,}000 \text{ ft} \bullet \text{lb}}{5 \text{ sec}}$$
$$P = 200 \text{ ft} \bullet \text{lb/sec}$$

The power involved with the elbow flexion exercises presented depends upon how fast the exercise was performed. If the work done during the single pulley exercise (26.67 ft • lb) is performed in 3 sec, then the power output for one repetition would be

$$P = \frac{W}{t}$$
$$P = \frac{26.67 \text{ ft} \bullet \text{lb}}{3 \text{ sec}}$$
$$P = 8.89 \text{ ft} \bullet \text{lb/sec}$$

Three sets of 10 repetitions would be 30 times 8.89 ft • lb/sec or 266.7 ft • lb/sec. If the exercise is performed so that each elbow flexion movement occurs in 1 sec, then the power output will be 3 times greater. For one repetition, the power output will be 26.67 ft • lb/sec, or 800.1 ft • lb/sec for 3 sets of 10 repetitions.

Power is an important aspect of everyday activities, in the workplace, and in sports performance. Walking, running, and climbing stairs require power to perform these tasks in a timely manner. More importantly, power is essential in preventing falls. Power production is related to the strength of a muscle, but it is different in that, to produce a greater magnitude of power, the muscle must contract more rapidly. The ability to contract a muscle or muscles rapidly to correct one's balance may allow the individual to avoid injury. As an individual ages, both strength and power decline. However, the speed of muscle contraction appears to decrease faster than the muscle's ability to produce force. Thus, muscle power declines faster than muscle strength. Power should be monitored as an individual ages. In the performance of sporting skills, power is related to the abilities of running, jumping, kicking, and throwing. All of these activities require a rapid application of force to be relatively successful.

Power training must involve force applied at a high velocity. For the lower limbs, power training has included rapid stair climbing, stair climbing with a weighted vest, rapid leg press, jumping rope, and vertical jumps. Power training for the upper limbs has included rapid bench

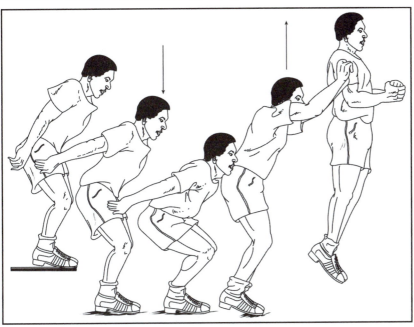

Figure 6-17. Plyometrics as one lands from a jump and jumps again.

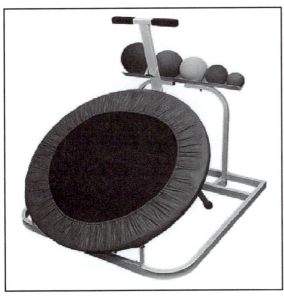

Figure 6-18. Upper limb plyometrics with a ball and mini-trampoline. Reprinted with permission from Patterson Medical/Sammons Preston, Bolingbrook, IL.

press, weighted ball with mini-trampoline, and rapid weightlifting. The loads for such activities vary, but the load for peak power is about 50% to 70% of 1 Repetition Maximum (1RM) for the lower limbs and 40% to 60% for the upper limbs.

Plyometrics is a training technique using the stretch-shorten cycle process of the muscles. An eccentric contraction followed quickly by a rapid concentric contraction provides a training stimulus for power for either lower or upper limbs. Jumping from a step, a squat, followed by a rapid jump is an example of plyometrics for the lower limbs (Figure 6-17). Catching a weighted ball and quickly throwing it provides a plyometric activity for the upper limbs (Figure 6-18). Plyometric training is recommended for injury prevention, later stages of rehabilitation, and special skill enhancement.

Activities

1. Define motion, dynamics, displacement, velocity, acceleration, and radian.
2. Show and describe the relationship between linear and angular motion.
3. Differentiate between kinematics and kinetics.
4. Provide and discuss examples of the effects of motion in the body, in clinical use, and in everyday activities.
5. Differentiate between centrifugal force and centripetal force.
6. Provide and discuss examples of kinetic approaches to evaluate forces in the body, in clinical use, and in everyday activities.
7. Relate the concepts of impulse and momentum.
8. Relate the concepts of work, energy, and power.
9. Discuss the importance of the fact that, in exercise, more force is needed to move a weight rapidly.
10. Discuss why athletes and patients are taught to roll when they fall?
11. Compare the processes of direct dynamics and inverse dynamics.
12. Discuss the importance of moment of inertia and radius of gyration in the design of prosthetics and orthotics.
13. Describe how sprinting can cause quadriceps and hamstring muscle strains.
14. If the force is equal, does an injury from rapid motion cause more, less, or the same damage as an injury occurring during a slower motion?
15. An upper limb 28 inches in length moves through an arc of 30 degrees in 0.75 sec. Assume that the limb does not bend during this motion.
    a. What is the average angular velocity of the limb in radians?
    b. What is the average linear velocity of a weight in the hand 26 in from the shoulder axis?
    c. What is the average linear velocity of the elbow 12 in from the shoulder axis?
16. Convert 30 degrees, 45 degrees, 60 degrees, 90 degrees, and 180 degrees to radians.
17. How much work does an individual do when lifting a 50-lb box from the ground onto a loading dock that is 2.5 ft high? What would be the power output if the box were lifted in 2 sec?
18. How much work does an individual do when sliding a 50-lb box up a 20-degree ramp ($\mu=0.3$) to the surface of the loading dock 2.5 ft high? What is the length of the surface of the ramp?
19. Compare the work sliding the box with lifting the box in the preceding problems. Would the coefficient of friction need to be more or less for the work in questions 17 and 18 to be equal?
20. Because strength training is angle specific, which exercise is better for functional activities of the knee: sitting using cuff weights or a semi-squat with a barbell? Explain.
21. Explain the concept of plyometric exercise.
22. Describe at least 2 methods of plyometric training.

Answers

14. An injury from rapid motion is more damaging because it involves more energy.
15. 0.70 rad/sec; 18.15 in/sec; 8.38 in/sec
16. 0.524; 0.785; 1.047; 1.57; 3.14
17. 125 ft • lb; 625 ft • lb/sec
18. 227 ft • lb; 7.3 ft
19. less

Suggested Reading

Alimusaj M, Fradet L, Braatz F, Gerner HJ, Wolf SI. Kinematics and kinetics with an adaptive ankle foot system during stair ambulation of transtibial amputees. *Gait Posture.* 2009;30:356-363.

Amis AA, Dowson D, Wright V. Analysis of elbow forces due to high-speed forearm movements. *J Biomech.* 1980;13:825-831.

Biewener AA, Roberts TJ. Muscle and tendon contributions to force, work, and elastic energy savings: a comparative perspective. *Exerc Sport Sci Rev.* 2000;28:99-107.

Chambers HG, Sutherland DH. A practical guide to gait analysis. *J Am Acad Orthop Surg.* 2002;10:222-231.

Collinger JL, Boninger ML, Koontz AM, et al. Shoulder biomechanics during the push phase of wheelchair propulsion: a multisite study of persons with paraplegia. *Arch Phys Med Rehabil.* 2008;89:667-676.

Damavandi M, Farahpour N, Allard P. Determination of body segment masses and centers of mass using a force plate method in individuals of different morphology. *Med Eng Phys.* 2009;31(9):1187-1194.

De Witt JK, Hagan RD, Cromwell RL. The effect of increasing inertia upon vertical ground reaction forces and temporal kinematics during locomotion. *J Exp Biol.* 2008;211:1087-1092.

DeVita P, Hortobagyi T. Age causes a redistribution of joint torques and powers during gait. *J Appl Physiol.* 2000;88:1804-1811.

Dubowsky SR, Rasmussen J, Sisto SA, Langrana NA. Validation of a musculoskeletal model of wheelchair propulsion and its application to minimizing shoulder joint forces. *J Biomech.* 2008;41:2981-2988.

Dubowsky SR, Sisto SA, Langrana NA. Comparison of kinematics, kinetics, and EMG throughout wheelchair propulsion in able-bodied and persons with paraplegia: an integrative approach. *J Biomech Eng.* 2009;131:021015.

Feltner ME, Bishop EJ, Perez CM. Segmental and kinetic contributions in vertical jumps performed with and without an arm swing. *Res Q Exerc Sport.* 2004;75:216-230.

Fukashiro S, Hay DC, Nagano A. Biomechanical behavior of muscle-tendon complex during dynamic human movements. *J Appl Biomech.* 2006;22:131-147.

Gallo LM. Modeling of temporomandibular joint function using MRI and jaw-tracking technologies—mechanics. *Cells Tissues Organs.* 2005;180:54-68.

Gitter A, Czerniecki J, Meinders M. Effect of prosthetic mass on swing phase work during above-knee amputee ambulation. *Am J Phys Med Rehabil.* 1997;76:114-121.

Hafner BJ, Sanders JE, Czerniecki JM, Fergason J. Transtibial energy-storage-and-return prosthetic devices: a review of energy concepts and a proposed nomenclature. *J Rehabil Res Dev.* 2002;39:1-11.

Hass CJ, Schick EA, Tillman MD, Chow JW, Brunt D, Caraugh JH. Knee biomechanics during landings: comparison of pre- and postpubescent females. *Med Sci Sports Exerc.* 2005;37:100-107.

Hemmerich A, Brown H, Smith S, Marthandam SS, Wyss UP. Hip, knee, and ankle kinematics of high range of motion activities of daily living. *J Orthop Res.* 2006;24:770-771.

Henriksen M, Simonsen EB, Alkjaer T, et al. Increased joint loads during walking—a consequence of pain relief in knee osteoarthritis. *Knee.* 2006;13:445-450.

Huang YC, Harbst K, Kotajarvi B, et al. Effects of ankle-foot orthoses on ankle and foot kinematics in patient with ankle osteoarthritis. *Arch Phys Med Rehabil.* 2006;87:710-716.

Jaskolski A, Kisiel K, Adach Z, Jaskolska A. The influence of elbow joint angle on different phases of force development during maximal voluntary contraction. *Can J Appl Physiol.* 2000;25:453-465.

Kawakami Y, Kubo K, Kanehisa H, Fukunaga T. Effect of series elasticity on isokinetic torque-angle relationship in humans. *Eur J Appl Physiol.* 2002;87:381-387.

Kawakami Y, Muraoka T, Ito S, Kanehisa H, Fukunaga T. In vivo muscle fibre behaviour during counter-movement exercise in humans reveals a significant role for tendon elasticity. *J Physiol.* 2002;540:635-646.

Keller TS, Colloca CJ. A rigid body model of the dynamic posteroanterior motion response of the human lumbar spine. *J Manipulative Physiol Ther.* 2002;25:485-496.

Kitaoka HB, Crevoisier XM, Hansen D, Katajarvi B, Harbst K, Kaufman KR. Foot and ankle kinematics and ground reaction forces during ambulation. *Foot Ankle Int.* 2006;27:808-813.

Kitaoka HB, Crevoisier XM, Harbst K, Hansen D, Kotajarvi B, Kaufman K. The effect of custom-made braces for the ankle and hindfoot on ankle and foot kinematics and ground reaction forces. *Arch Phys Med Rehabil.* 2006;87:130-135.

Koolstra JH. Dynamics of the human masticatory system. *Crit Rev Oral Biol Med.* 2002;13:366-376.

Lafortune MA, Cavanagh PR, Sommer HJ 3rd, Kalenak A. Foot inversion-eversion and knee kinematics during walking. *J Orthop Res.* 1994;12:412-420.

Lenaerts G, Bartels W, Gelaude F, et al. Subject-specific hip geometry and hip joint centre location affects calculated contact forces at the hip during gait. *J Biomech.* 2009;42:1246-1251.

Li G, Pierce JE, Herndon JH. A global optimization method for prediction of muscle forces of human musculoskeletal system. *J Biomech.* 2006;39:522-529.

Liu Y, Peng CH, Wei SH, Chi JC, Tsai FR, Chen JY. Active leg stiffness and energy stored in the muscles during maximal counter movement jump in the aged. *J Electromyogr Kinesiol.* 2006;16:342-351.

Martin PE, Cavanagh PR. Segment interactions within the swing leg during unloaded and loaded running. *J Biomech.* 1990;23:529-536.

Mason JJ, Leszko F, Johnson T, Komistek RD. Patellofemoral joint forces. *J Biomech.* 2008;41:2337-2348.

McBride JM, McCaulley GO, Cormie P. Influence of preactivity and eccentric muscle activity on concentric performance during vertical jumping. *J Strength Cond Res.* 2008;22:750-757.

Morrow MM, Hurd WJ, Kaufman KR, An KN. Shoulder demands in manual wheelchair users across a spectrum of activities. *J Electromyogr Kinesiol.* 2009;20(1):61-67.

Olney SJ, Griffin MP, Monga TN, McBride ID. Work and power in gait of stroke patients. *Arch Phys Med Rehabil.* 1991;72:309-314.

Ounpuu S. The biomechanics of walking and running. *Clin Sports Med.* 1994;13:843-863.

Pal S, Langenderfer JE, Stowe JQ, Laz PJ, Petrella AJ, Rullkoetter PJ. Probabilistic modeling of knee muscle moment arms: effects of methods, origin-insertion, and kinematic variability. *Ann Biomed Eng.* 2007;35:1632-1642.

Pataky TC, Zatsiorsky VM, Challis JH. A simple method to determine body segment masses in vivo: reliability, accuracy and sensitivity analysis. *Clin Biomech (Bristol, Avon).* 2003;18:364-368.

Patel VV, Hall K, Ries M, et al. Magnetic resonance imaging of patellofemoral kinematics with weight-bearing. *J Bone Joint Surg Am.* 2003;85-A:2419-2424.

Piriyaprasarth P, Morris ME. Psychometric properties of measurement tools for quantifying knee joint position and movement: a systematic review. *Knee.* 2007;14:2-8.

Prince F, Winter DA, Sjonnensen G, Powell C, Wheeldon RK. Mechanical efficiency during gait of adults with transtibial amputation: a pilot study comparing the SACH, Seattle, and Golden-Ankle prosthetic feet. *J Rehabil Res Dev.* 1998;35:177-185.

Protopapadaki A, Drechsler WI, Cramp MC, Coutts FJ, Scott OM. Hip, knee, ankle kinematics and kinetics during stair ascent and descent in healthy young individuals. *Clin Biomech (Bristol, Avon).* 2007;22:203-210.

Reinbolt JA, Haftka RT, Chmielewski TL, Fregly BJ. Are patient-specific joint and inertial parameters necessary for accurate inverse dynamics analyses of gait? *IEEE Trans Biomed Eng.* 2007;54:782-793.

Reisman M, Burdett RG, Simon SR, Norkin C. Elbow moment and forces at the hands during swing-through axillary crutch gait. *Phys Ther.* 1985;65:601-605.

Romo HD. Specialized prostheses for activities. An update. *Clin Orthop Relat Res.* 1999;(361):63-70.

Rundquist PJ, Anderson DD, Guanche CA, Ludewig PM. Shoulder kinematics in subjects with frozen shoulder. *Arch Phys Med Rehabil.* 2003;84:1473-1479.

Sasso RC, Best NM. Cervical kinematics after fusion and bryan disc arthroplasty. *J Spinal Disord Tech.* 2008;21:19-22.

Schache AG, Baker R. On the expression of joint moments during gait. *Gait Posture.* 2007;25:440-452.

Schmitz A, Silder A, Heiderscheit B, Mahoney J, Thelen DG. Differences in lower-extremity muscular activation during walking between healthy older and young adults. *J Electromyogr Kinesiol.* 2008;19(6):1085-1091.

Selles RW, Bussmann JB, Wagenaar RC, Stam HJ. Effects of prosthetic mass and mass distribution on kinematics and energetics of prosthetic gait: a systematic review. *Arch Phys Med Rehabil.* 1999;80:1593-1599.

Seth A, Pandy MG. A neuromusculoskeletal tracking method for estimating individual muscle forces in human movement. *J Biomech.* 2007;40:356-366.

Siegel KL, Kepple TM, Stanhope SJ. Joint moment control of mechanical energy flow during normal gait. *Gait Posture.* 2004;19:69-75.

Silder A, Heiderscheit B, Thelen DG. Active and passive contributions to joint kinetics during walking in older adults. *J Biomech.* 2008;41:1520-1527.

Silder A, Whittington B, Heiderscheit B, Thelen DG. Identification of passive elastic joint moment-angle relationships in the lower extremity. *J Biomech.* 2007;40:2628-2635.

Stockbrugger BA, Haennel RG. Validity and reliability of a medicine ball explosive power test. *J Strength Cond Res.* 2001;15: 431-438.

Teixeira LF, Olney SJ. Relationship between alignment and kinematic and kinetic measures of the knee of osteoarthritic elderly subjects in level walking. *Clin Biomech (Bristol, Avon).* 1996;11:126-134.

Tillman MD, Hass CJ, Chow JW, Brunt D. Lower extremity coupling parameters during locomotion and landings. *J Appl Biomech.* 2005;21:359-370.

Toumi H, Best TM, Martin A, F'Guyer S, Poumarat G. Effects of eccentric phase velocity of plyometric training on the vertical jump. *Int J Sports Med.* 2004;25:391-398.

Tsirakos D, Baltzopoulos V, Bartlett R. Inverse optimization: functional and physiological considerations related to the force-sharing problem. *Crit Rev Biomed Eng.* 1997;25:371-407.

Versluys R, Beyl P, Van Damme M, Desomer A, Van Ham R, Lefeber D. Prosthetic feet: state-of-the-art review and the importance of mimicking human ankle-foot biomechanics. *Disabil Rehabil Assist Technol.* 2009;4:65-75.

Whittington B, Silder A, Heiderscheit B, Thelen DG. The contribution of passive-elastic mechanisms to lower extremity joint kinetics during human walking. *Gait Posture.* 2008;27:628-634.

Wilson JM, Flanagan EP. The role of elastic energy in activities with high force and power requirements: a brief review. *J Strength Cond Res.* 2008;22:1705-1715.

Yang JJ, Feng X, Xiang Y, Kim JH, Rajulu S. Determining the three-dimensional relation between the skeletal elements of the human shoulder complex. *J Biomech.* 2009;42:1762-1767.

chapter 7

Application

Objectives

1. Define stability, balance, and posture.
2. Differentiate among stable, unstable, and neutral equilibrium.
3. Describe how stability of an object depends upon 4 characteristics.
4. Present and explain clinical and everyday life examples of stability and balance.
5. Locate the center of mass for a specific posture from a picture.
6. Locate the center of mass for an individual's total body.
7. Locate the center of mass or determine the weight of an individual's body segment.
8. Describe the characteristics of a good measuring instrument.
9. Evaluate the characteristics of a specific measuring instrument.
10. Describe the specific factors involved in determining muscle strength.
11. Evaluate and compare devices and activities used to strengthen muscles.
12. Describe methods to analyze human motion.
13. Relate mechanics to gait and locomotion.

Introduction

In previous chapters, we have seen how to approach examples of static and dynamic equilibrium. By using these basic techniques, an endless number of problems can be attacked. In this chapter, a few selected examples and problems relating to body mechanics, exercise programs, and other clinical approaches are presented.

It must be remembered that when we select static positions for analysis, we are only approximating the precise forces accompanying actual movement. Analysis by this means ignores co-contractions, accelerations, momentum, and frictional effects. However, the conditions under which very slow, deliberate movements common in therapeutic exercises are carried out resemble those of static postures. Thus, analysis of a series of selected positions will give a minimum approximation of required muscle tension and articular forces. Effects of non-contractile tissues and changing location of joint centers also reduce the accuracy of the computations. Thus, the problems presented in this chapter will not be exact, but will be somewhat simplified to show the general procedures for biomechanical analysis and approximate values that really exist.

LeVeau BF.
Biomechanics of Human Motion: Basics and Beyond for the Health Professions (pp 137-166).
© 2011 SLACK Incorporated

Stability and Balance

STABILITY

Stability can be defined as resistance to change. In mechanics, stability is defined as the resistance to change in position or equilibrium of an object or a body. The force of gravity can assist in maintaining stability or may assist in disruption of the position of an object. Often, external forces acting on the object tend to change the position or disrupt the equilibrium of the object.

An object is considered to be in stable equilibrium if a force displaces it slightly and the object returns to its original position. The object is difficult to displace. Figure 7-1A illustrates a stable object. The equilibrium of an object is unstable when it is slightly displaced by a force and the displacement continues to increase. The object is easy to displace. Figure 7-1B illustrates an unstable object. An object is in neutral equilibrium if it remains in its displaced position after a force slightly displaces it. Figure 7-1C shows an object that has neutral equilibrium.

The stability of an object depends upon 4 characteristics:

1. The mass of the object

2. The area of the object's base

3. The height of the object's center of mass

4. The location of the object's center of mass within its base of support.

The more stable object has a large mass, a large area for a base of support, and a low center of gravity located over the center of the base of support. The location of the center of mass of the object is a major determinant for its stability. If the center of mass is low and in the center of the base of support and the base of support is large, work must be done to lift the center of mass over the edge of the base of support in order to displace the object (Figure 7-2). Very little work is needed to displace an object if its center of mass is high and its base of support is small.

By increasing the weight of an object, we increase its stability. A heavier object, although it has the same dimensions, is more stable than a lighter object.

The moments of force acting on the object and the moment of the gravitational force on the object's center of mass contribute to the object's stability. In a stable object, the gravitational force moment acting on the center of mass tends to retard the displacement of the object. To displace the object, a moment of force acting to displace the object must be greater than the gravitational moment. However, once the center of mass and the line of application of the gravitational force fall outside of the object's base of support, gravity will begin to aid in displacing the object (Figure 7-3).

The stability of an object is indirectly proportional to the height of its center of mass above its base. An object with a very low center of mass is more stable than one with a high center of mass. The punching doll in Figure 7-4 is an example. Because of the heavy weight located at the base of the doll, its center of mass is quite low. As you hit the doll, it will be displaced, but it tends to return to its original position.

As an individual is standing with the feet together, the line of application of the gravitational force (line of gravity) falls anterior to the ankle joint over the center of the base of support. This location of the line of gravity is essential so that the chance of falling backwards is reduced. This location, however, produces a moment of force anterior to the ankle that requires continual contraction of the plantar flexor muscles to establish equilibrium around the ankle. The body has a sway back and forth over the base of support, but rarely moves posterior to the ankle joint. An individual has a larger base of support and more stability if the feet are moved apart with one slightly ahead of the other or an assistive device is used (Figure 7-5). Figure 7-6 illustrates stable and unstable positions while using crutches.

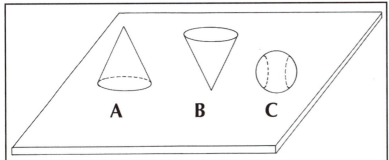

Figure 7-1. Stable, unstable, and neutral equilibrium. The cone in A is stable; the cone in B is unstable; and the ball in C is neutral.

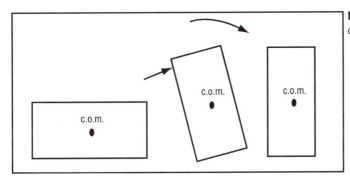

Figure 7-2. Work done to lift the center of mass over the edge.

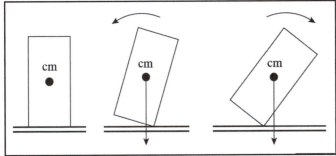

Figure 7-3. Relationship of center of mass to base of support. (A) The box is more stable when the center of mass is over the center of the base of support. (B) The box will fall backward to its stable position if the force is released. (C) If the center of mass goes beyond the base of support, the box will fall over.

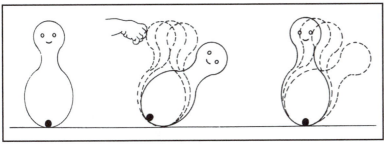

Figure 7-4. A punching doll with a low center of mass is difficult to tip over.

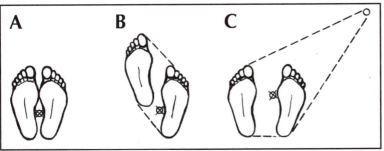

Figure 7-5. The position of the feet determines the size of the supporting area of the body. B has a larger supporting area than A. Use of a cane can greatly extend the base of support (C) and the area over which the body is stable.

Figure 7-6. Bases of support with varying degrees of stability. In A and B, the patient has a large base of support. The position in C provides more stability in the frontal plane than in the sagittal plane.

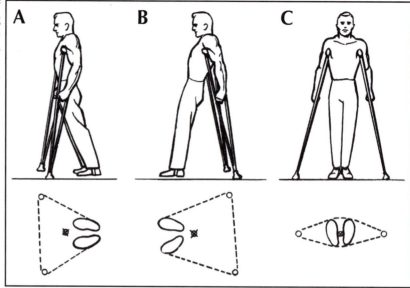

BALANCE

Balance is directly related to stability. We can define balance as the ability to maintain the center of mass over the base of support. Balancing one's body may range from performing a one-hand stand on parallel bars (Figure 7-7), standing on a balance beam (Figure 7-8), maintaining sitting balance (Figure 7-9), or resisting from being pushed over while in the quadriped position (Figure 7-10). For each of these positions, the center of mass of the entire body must be over the base of support. The center of mass is not located anterior to the sacrum (S_2) for each of these positions. Each body part, or segment, contributes to the location of the total center of mass.

The upright human body is least stable when an individual is standing on one foot (Figure 7-11), during single limb support of gait and stair climbing, or when dressing. Individuals with balance problems must adjust their approach to these postures to prevent a fall in such unstable situations. Assistive devices can enlarge the base of support and provide a third or fourth point for stability (see Figures 7-5 and 7-6). Holding onto a handrail provides a moment of force that enhances one's balance while traversing stairs. Sitting lowers the center of mass and increases the size of the base of support for dressing activities.

POSTURE AND CENTER OF MASS

The force exerted by an object as a result of gravitational pull may be considered as a single force representing the sum of all of the little individual weights within the object. The magnitude of the single resultant force will equal the combined individual weights of the component units of the object. The line of application of the resultant force will pass through a point about which all of the moments of the individual weights on one side will be exactly equal to the combined individual moments on the other side of the point.

Posture is the position of the body brought about by the arrangement of the individual body segments for a specific purpose. Most commonly, we think of posture being an upright stance with the feet together and the body in a relaxed position. However, any body position can be considered a posture for a given activity. A change in the posture from the relaxed upright position requires that the individual body segments be moved. Such movement of the individual segments affects the balance and stability of the body.

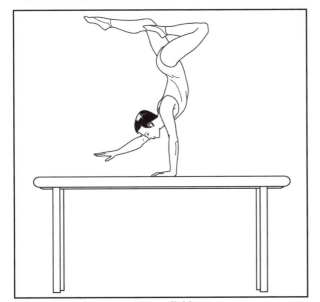

Figure 7-7. Balance on the parallel bars.

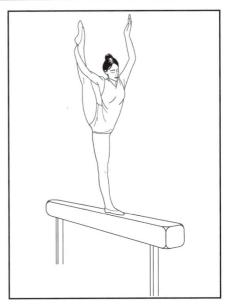

Figure 7-8. Balance on the balance beam.

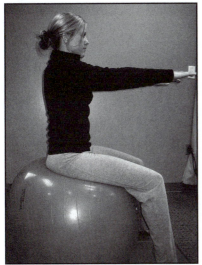

Figure 7-9. Sitting balance on a ball.

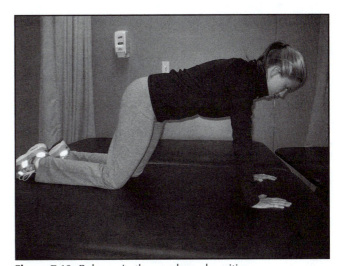

Figure 7-10. Balance in the quadruped position.

In certain postures, the center of mass may lie in space outside of the body itself. When a person leans forward to pick up an object from the floor, his or her center of mass may be displaced to a point anterior to the trunk (although it is still over the feet). The center of mass also moves forward when one is in a sitting position. Compare the areas of the base of support for conventional straight chairs and wheelchairs. Note that wheelchairs are designed for maximum stability. Patients with lower limb amputations have a higher center of mass, and when they are on crutches or in a wheelchair, their balance will be less stable. In some cases, adjustments to the wheelchair may be necessary (Figure 7-12).

The location of the center of mass of the body and its relationship to the base of support for any posture can be determined by summing the product of the weight (W_1) times the center of mass (x1) for each individual segment ($W_1 \times x_1$). The total moment (W x x) of the body weight

Figure 7-11. Balance standing on one foot.

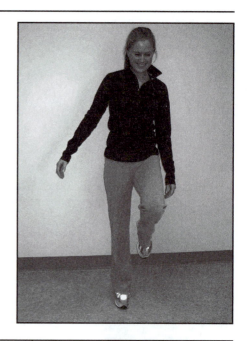

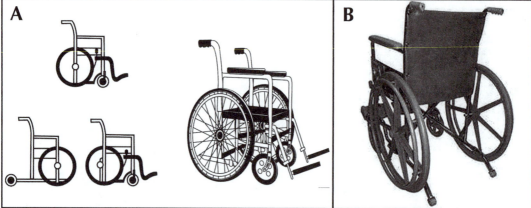

Figure 7-12. (A) Adjustment for wheelchair bases. (B) Universal Fit Adjustable Anti-Tippers, TuffCare Wheelchair Accessory Bolt-On Anti-Tipper. Reprinted with permission from Patterson Medical/Sammons Preston, Bolingbrook, IL.

(W) times the location of its center of mass in the x-direction (x) equals the sum of the moments of all of the separate body segments (eg, foot, leg, thigh, hand, forearm, etc). The same relationship exists for the total moment in the y-direction. The location of x and y define the location of the center of mass for the entire body.

$$Wx = W_1x_1 + W_2x_2 + W_3x_3 + \ldots$$
$$W = W_1 + W_2 + W_3 + \ldots$$
$$x = \frac{(W_1x_1 + W_2x_2 + W_3x_3 + \ldots)}{(W_1 + W_2 + W_3 + \ldots)}$$
$$Wy = W_1y_1 + W_2y_2 + W_3y_3 + \ldots$$
$$W = W_1 + W_2 + W_3 + \ldots$$
$$y = \frac{(W_1y_1 + W_2y_2 + W_3y_3 + \ldots)}{(W_1 + W_2 + W_3 + \ldots)}$$

The location of the center of mass of the body taken from a picture for any posture can be determined using these equations and an x-y coordinate system. The center of mass of a combination of segments (such as the hand, forearm, and arm) may be determined in a similar manner. The total moment for the combined segments (W_t x x_t) equals the sum of the moments of the individual segments (W_1 x x_1 + W_2 x x_2 + W_3 x x_3 + ...) in the x-direction and (W_t x y_t) equals the sum of the moments of the individual segments (W_1 x y_1 + W_2 x y_2 + W_3 x y_3 + ...) in the y-direction.

BOARD AND SCALE METHOD

To determine the location of the center of mass for the entire body, the board and scale method may be used (Figure 7-13). The materials needed to perform this task are a board large enough for an individual to lay on (approximately 3 ft x 7 ft), 2 3-ft long sharp-edged boards (1 in x 1 in), a scale to determine weight, and a block of wood of sufficient size to fit under one of the sharp-edge boards (4 in x 4 in x 3 ft long). The specific procedure is as follows:

1. Place the large board horizontally on the 2 sharp-edge supports, one at each end.
2. Have one sharp-edge support resting on the center of the scale platform and the other support on the wooden block so that the large board is level.
3. Take a reading from the scale (S_o) to be subtracted from later readings and eliminating the effect of the board.
4. Measure the distance between the sharp-edge supports (d).
5. For ease of calculation, have the subject lie supine on the board with the soles of the feet directly above the sharp edge on the wooden block and the head toward the scale end of the board.
6. Take the scale reading (S_1). The effect of the body is $S_1 - S_o$.
7. Use the second condition of equilibrium to determine the distance the center of mass (d_1) is away from the soles of the feet.

$$\Sigma M = 0$$
$$(W \times d_1) - [(S_1 - S_o) \times d)] = 0$$
$$(W \times d_1) = [(S_1 - S_o) \times d)]$$
$$d_1 = \frac{[(S_1 - S_o) \times d)]}{W}$$

8. Measure d_1 from the soles of the feet toward the head to locate the height of the center of mass of the body.

Figure 7-13 shows a 160-lb person lying supine on a board with 72 in between the supports with a scale value of ($S_1 - S_o$) 80 lb. The location of the center of gravity is calculated to be 36 in above the feet.

To find the anterior-posterior (sagittal plane) and the lateral (frontal plane) locations of the center of mass using a smaller board (3 ft x 3 ft), repeat the board and scale procedures (measure from appropriate body landmark) with the subject standing. For the anterior-posterior location, have the subject face the scale end. For the lateral location, the subject should have one side toward the scale.

SEGMENT CENTER OF MASS AND WEIGHT

Determining the weight of a body segment makes use of the board and scale method (Figure 7-14). This procedure separates the segment weight (W_1) from the total body weight (W).

Figure 7-13. Board and scale method. Method of locating the body's center of mass between the soles of the feet and crown of the head.

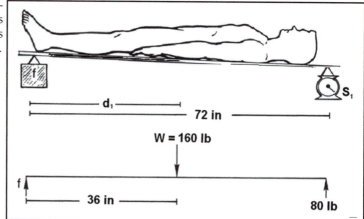

Figure 7-14. Method of weighing body segments with board and scale.

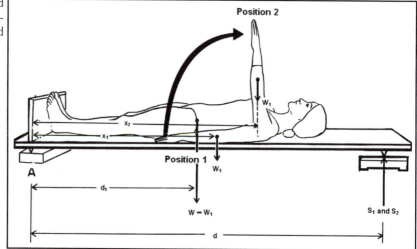

The estimated location of the center of mass of the segment must be located. The specific procedure using the upper limb as an example is as follows:

1. Perform steps 1 through 7 listed in the board and scale method to locate the center of mass for the entire body. (Record S_o, d, S_1, W, d_1.)
2. Measure the horizontal distance from the estimated center of mass of the upper limb to the sharp edge on the wooden block (x_1).
3. Flex the shoulder to 90 degrees, raising it to a vertical position.
4. Take the scale reading (S_2).
5. Measure the horizontal distance from the estimated center of mass of the upper limb to the sharp edge on the wooden block (x_2).
6. Use the principle of moments to determine the weight of the limb. (S_o is not needed for this calculation.)

$$S_1 \times d = (W_1 \times x_1) + [(W - W_1) \times d_1]$$
$$S_2 \times d = (W_1 \times x_2) + [(W - W_1) \times d_1]$$

Subtract the first equation from the second equation.

$$(S_2 - S_1) \times d = W_1 \times (x_2 - x_1)$$
$$W_1 = \frac{[(S_2 - S_1) * d]}{(x_2 - x_1)}$$

The weight of the upper limb segment is W_1. Other body segments may be determined using this same procedure if they can be measured so that the center of mass is located directly above the joint (x_2). The center of mass of the segment $(x_2 - x_1)$ may be located by the same equation

$$(x_2 - x_1) = \frac{(S_2 - S_1) \times d}{W_1}$$

$$x_1 = x_2 - \frac{(S_2 - S_1) \times d}{W_1}$$

Factors in Recording Muscle Strength

Anyone dealing with exercise training should know the biomechanical factors involved in the evaluation of muscular strength. This information has been presented in the previous chapters and will be summarized in this section.

MEASURING INSTRUMENTS

An important aspect of evaluation of strength is the criteria of a good measuring instrument or testing device (Table 7-1). A test that does not meet these criteria is of questionable value. A test should be selected that meets the criteria.

The instrument must be able to discriminate or determine differences among levels of strength. The manual muscle test determines the difference whether a muscle has no activity, whether the muscle can overcome a great amount of resistance, or whether the muscle has 3 levels of contractile ability in between.

The instrument must be able to be quantifiable or provide numerical values for the level of strength. The numbers provided should be in a ratio level of measurement rather than interval, ordinal, or nominal. Most often, grades for strength evaluation using a manual muscle test are recorded as numerical scores ranging from zero (0) to five (5).

The instrument must be reliable and must provide the same value when measured more than once. If it is not reliable, it cannot be valid, and it must be a valid measure. An instrument claiming to measure muscle strength must measure muscle strength.

The procedures for the use of the measuring instrument must be standardized so that the test is administered in the same manner each time it is used. The test should be easy to administer and must not be time consuming (economy of time). Normative data should be available so that the results of an individual can be compared to others.

BIOMECHANICAL FACTORS

When evaluating an individual's muscle strength, we must realize that the strength of the muscle or muscle group is being evaluated indirectly. The measuring instrument is not attached directly to the muscle or tendon, but a lever system is used to determine the magnitude of the muscle force. The instrument is determining the magnitude of force at its point of application that is related to the magnitude of the muscle force. This indirect evaluation is influenced by biomechanical factors, such as body position and type of contraction (Table 7-2).

Body Position

The position of the body part involved in the evaluation of muscle strength plays a major role in determining muscle force (Figure 7-15). The force of gravity acting on the body part, the angle of the line of application with the body part, the effective length of the lever arm resisting the muscle force (point of application of the testing instrument), the length of the muscle, and stabilization of the body part all affect the determination of the magnitude of muscle force.

TABLE 7-1

Criteria of Measurement Instrument

• Ability to descriminate	• Standardized
• Quantifiable	• Ease of administration
• Reliable	• Economy of time
• Valid	• Availability of norms

TABLE 7-2

Factors Influencing Recorded Strength Values

I.   Body position
II. Type of contraction
III. Other
       Physiological
       Psychological

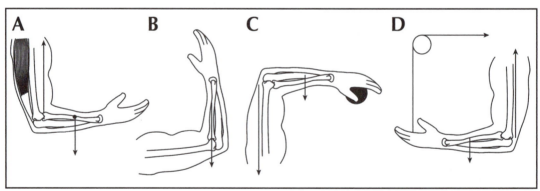

Figure 7-15. Effect of gravity acting on the forearm muscles. (A) Elbow flexor muscles must overcome the weight of the limb. (B) When the center of mass of the body part passes through the joint axis, it produces no moment around the joint. (C) Elbow extensors must overcome the weight of the limb and load. (D) Gravity is assisting the elbow extensor muscles.

The force of gravity acting on the body part basically refers to the weight of the body part. The rotatory effect of the force of gravity is greatest when the body part is horizontal (Figure 7-15A) and least when the body part is vertical with the center of mass directly above the axis of motion (Figure 7-15B). The body part may be in a position that adds resistance to the muscle force (Figure 7-15C) or in a position that assists the muscle force (Figure 7-15D). If the body part moves through a range of motion during the testing procedure, the body part will provide a variable resistance to the muscle force.

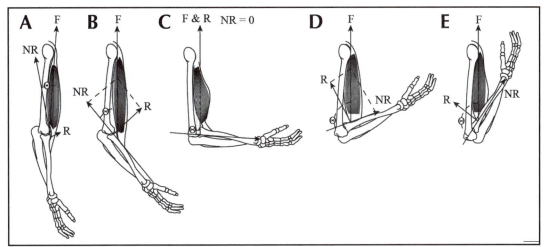

Figure 7-16. The rotatory force component of the muscle increases as the elbow flexes to 90 degrees where it becomes maximum. As the elbow continues to flex, the rotator component decreases.

The angle of the line of application of the muscle force influences the amount of rotatory force available to be recorded by a testing instrument (Figure 7-16). The maximum rotatory force occurs when the muscle's line of application is perpendicular (90 degrees) to the body part. The rotatory force is least when the muscle's line of application is nearly parallel to the body part (Figure 7-16A, E). The actual magnitude of the muscle force can only be determined if the angle for the line of application is known.

The point of application of the measuring instrument in relation to the axis of motion provides the lever arm length that opposes the muscle moment (torque). If the measuring instrument is located close to the axis of motion, the measuring instrument will reveal a greater magnitude than when the measuring instrument is located at a greater distance away from the axis of motion (Figure 7-17).

The length of the contracting muscle affects the magnitude of force it produces. In general, a muscle that is in a lengthened position will produce a greater force than a muscle that is shortened (Figure 7-18). When testing a 2- or multi-joint muscle, the position of all of the involved joints must be considered.

The stability of the body part being tested is also important. The adjacent body segments must provide a stable base for the segment involved in the testing. An unstable segment will allow inaccurate results from unwanted motion, muscle substitution, and improper positioning.

Type of Contraction

The type and speed of contraction influence the value obtained for the magnitude of muscle force (Figure 7-19). Less magnitude of force is recorded for a muscle that is contracting concentrically (shortening). The faster the muscle contracts concentrically, the less will be the recorded strength of the muscle (Figure 7-20). A greater magnitude of force is recorded from a muscle that is contracting isometrically (no external motion) than one that is contracting concentrically. The greatest magnitude of force is recorded from a muscle that is contracting eccentrically (lengthening). Note that the recording values are different, but the force produced by the actual muscle activity may not be that different. You must remember the resisting inertia involved in a moving object, ma and $I\alpha$.

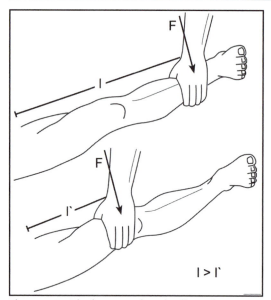

Figure 7-17. The lever arm length affects the magnitude of force recorded by a measuring device.

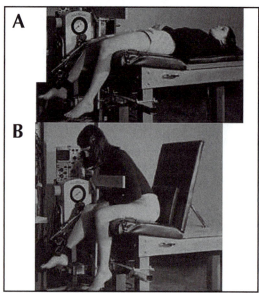

Figure 7-18. Effect of muscle length. (A) Hamstring muscles in a lengthened position produce more force than (B) muscles that are in a shortened position. (Reprinted from Lunnen JD, Yack J, LeVeau BF. Relationship between muscle length muscle action potential, and torque of the hamstring muscles. *Physical Therapy.* 1981;61:190-195, with permission of the American Physical Therapy Association. This material is copyrighted, and any further reproduction or distribution is prohibited.)

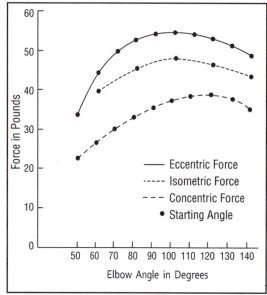

Figure 7-19. Curves of maximum eccentric, isometric, and concentric forces of forearm flexors. (Reprinted with permission from the American Physiological Society. Figure 2 from M. Singh and P. V. Karpovich. Isotonic and isometric forces of forearm flexors and extensors. *J Appl Physiol.* 21(4):1435-1437, 1966.)

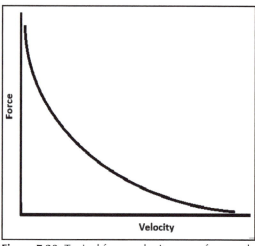

Figure 7-20. Typical force-velocity curve for muscle contraction. With a greater velocity of contraction, less measureable force is present. (Adapted from Komi PV. Measurement of the force-velocity relationship in human muscle under concentric and eccentric contractions. In Cerquiglini S, Venerando S, Wartenweiler J, eds. *Biomechanics III.* Baltimore, MD: University Park Press; 1973:227.)

Other

Co-contraction of antagonistic muscles will reduce the magnitude of the recorded force. The muscle being tested may be producing a large magnitude of force, but this magnitude will not be recorded if the antagonist muscles are active.

Joint limitations, such as friction, bony mechanical block, muscle tightness, and pain, will also affect the recorded force values.

Other non-biomechanical factors should also be considered during muscle strength testing and training. These include warm-up, learning trials, motivation, rest between trials, and age and gender of the individual.

Analysis of Exercise Method

Biomechanical factors used to measure muscle strength are also involved in exercises used to maintain or improve strength. Anyone who considers themselves knowledgeable in the science of exercise must be able to analyze activities and devices used in strength training.

When deciding which exercise mode to use, the most important concern is the desired result of the activity. The effects of strength training are highly specific. Specificity of training refers to the concept that the muscle adapts specifically to the type of training performed. Biomechanically, muscle adaptation to training involves the muscle or muscle group trained, the amount of resistance (load), the range of motion or specificity of the angle being exercised (displacement), type of muscle contraction (concentric, eccentric, or isometric), the speed of the movement (power), and the rate of force development (impulse). The second condition of equilibrium ($\Sigma M = 0$) must be involved in any analysis of a strength training activity. The distance that the point of application of the load is from the axis of motion (d) establishes the lever length for the moment (L x d) developed by the load (L). These concepts have been presented earlier. In the following paragraphs, some specific procedures and devices will be analyzed related to their specificity for training strength.

GRAVITY RESISTANCE

All exercise devices use some type of force to provide resistance to the muscle contraction. The force of gravity is the most common force to be used as a load for strength training. A body part (segment or combined segments), cuff weights, dumbbells, a barbell and plates, or a box offer a point of application on the body, a vertical line of application, a downward direction, and a selected magnitude of force.

Body Segment

When using a body segment as a load, the center of mass of the segment is the point of application, and magnitude of the load is the weight of the segment or combined segments. Almost any segment or combination of segments may be used as the load.

Example

For strengthening of the abdominal muscles (Figure 7-21), the segments of the head, arms, and trunk are the load. The weight of these body segments does not change, but the resisting moment can be changed by changing the position of the arms. In general, the further the arms are moved away from the hips, the greater the resisting moment will be. The moment set up by the center of mass is less when the arms are at the side of the trunk (Figure 7-21A); it is greater when the arms are across the chest (Figure 7-21B); and is greater still if the arms are over the head (Figure 7-21C). The position of the combined segments also affects the load (Figure 7-22).

Figure 7-21. The lever arm of gravitational force (W) is increased by moving the arms upward (lever arm d″ > d′ > d).

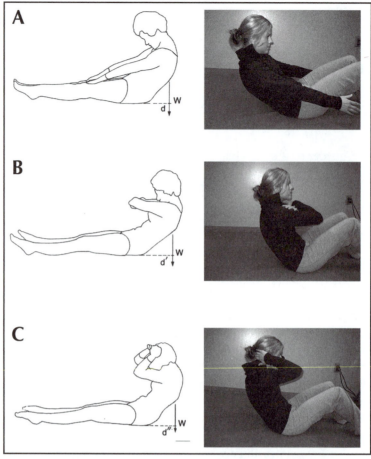

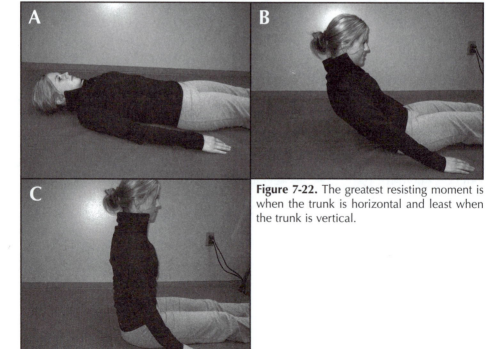

Figure 7-22. The greatest resisting moment is when the trunk is horizontal and least when the trunk is vertical.

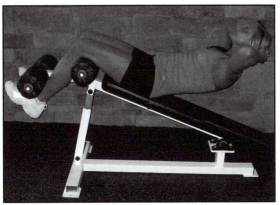

Figure 7-23. Inclined sit-up.

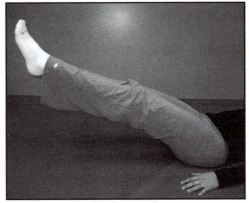

Figure 7-24. Double leg raise.

When the trunk is nearly horizontal without touching the floor or mat, the resisting moment is greatest. When the trunk is vertical, the resisting moment is least (maybe zero). In between the horizontal and vertical positions, the load changes in relationship to the cosine of the angle of the trunk with the horizontal or sine of the angle of the gravity line of application with the trunk (resolution of forces). To change the resisting moment, weights may be added to the hands, or the body position may be inclined on an inclined bench with the head up or the head down (Figure 7-23). The exercise may be performed through a large range of motion (horizontal to vertical) or through a small range (to when the scapulae leave the mat). The motion can emphasize concentric and eccentric without an isometric phase, or it may be predominantly isometric. The exercise may emphasize speed of movement by performing as many as possible in 1 minute, or it may be held isometrically for several seconds. The concentric contraction may be explosive or begin at a very slow rate. The activity is mainly limited by the line of application. Raising or lowering the lower limbs can also provide a load to the abdominal muscles (Figure 7-24). For exercises of the abdominal muscles, be aware of what is occurring in the lumbar spine.

External Load

An external load, such as cuff weights, dumbbells, a barbell and plates, or a box, add a load to the body segment or segments. The point of application of the additional load is in the hands or wherever the load attaches to the body. The line of application is vertical, and the direction is down. The magnitude of the load can be adjusted to the ability of the individual and the purpose of the exercise. The load may be moved through a large range of motion concentrically and eccentrically or be held in one position isometrically. Remember that, as the body part moves through the range of motion (Figure 7-25), the resisting moments will change in relationship to the cosine of the angle of the body part with the horizontal or sine of the angle of the gravity line of application with the body part (resolution of forces). The angle of the muscle line of application and the length of the muscle will likely change as well.

Example

For strengthening the quadriceps muscles, cuff weights may be used. With the individual sitting and the legs over the edge of the treatment table, a cuff weight is attached to the ankle. The combined segments of the leg and foot and the cuff weights provide the load to the quadriceps muscles. The external load may be changed by using a different cuff weight. Usually, this exercise travels concentrically from 90 degrees of knee flexion to full extension (0 degrees) and

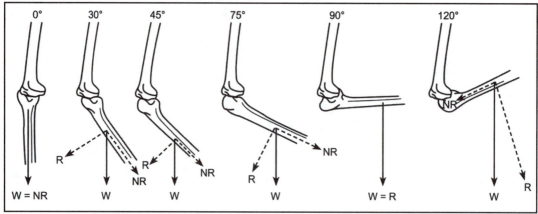

Figure 7-25. The change in gravitational components of the forearm as it moves through the range of motion.

eccentrically back to 90 degrees. The motion can emphasize concentric and eccentric without an isometric phase, or it may be predominantly isometric in full extension (0 degrees). The exercise may emphasize speed of movement by performing repetitions as quickly as possible, or it may be held isometrically for several seconds. The concentric contraction may be explosive or begin at a very slow rate. The resisting moments at 90 degrees with the load directly below the knee will be zero. Such a situation places an increased load on the collateral ligaments of the knee. As the knee is extended, the resisting moments increase until the leg is horizontal where the resisting moments are maximum (Figure 7-26). The activity is mainly limited by the line of application of the load. Partial squatting with a barbell held in the hands as a load will also provide resistance for the quadriceps muscles (Figure 7-27). In this situation, however, the greatest resisting moment is when the knee is flexed and is near zero when the knees are extended. Using the barbell provides a bilateral exercise, while the cuff weight is done unilaterally. For exercise of the quadriceps muscles, be aware of what is occurring at the patellofemoral joint (composition of forces).

Pulley Weights

Exercise devices using pulleys or pulleys and levers with plates as resistance are quite common. The resisting force is gravity acting on the plates. The point of application is the point of contact of the pulley or lever handle on the body part. These devices have plates as the resisting load. A major difference with this type of device compared to the other gravity devices is that the cord in the pulley system changes the line of application and direction of the resisting force. The line of application is not always vertical, and the direction is not always down. When analyzing the pulley device, the cord establishes the line of application, and the direction is traced through the cord away from the point of application. The motion usually is concentric and eccentric without an isometric phase, but it may include an isometric phase. Several variables can exist using this type of device. As the body part moves through the range of motion, the pulley cord will change its angle with that body part. The greatest resisting load occurs when the line of application is perpendicular (90 degrees) with the body part. The effect of the load decreases as the angle changes from perpendicular. The pulley and lever system prevents this change in line of application by having the cord attached to a continuous lever (circle) that has an arm extended to the point of application on the body (Figure 7-28). With the cord attached to the lever system, the resisting moment of the plates attached to the cord remains constant.

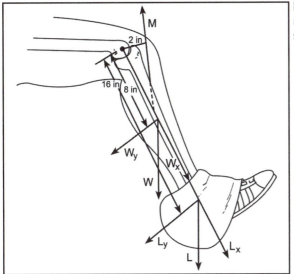

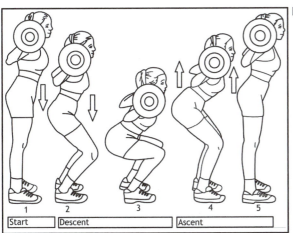

Figure 7-26. Force components and resisting moments (W_y x 8 and S_y x 16) for knee extension exercise.

Figure 7-27. Squat with a barbell.

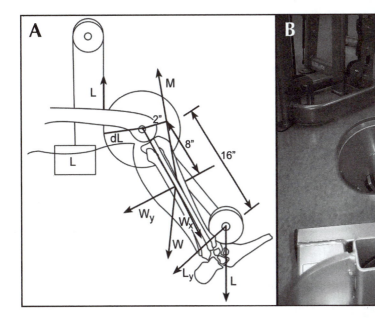

Figure 7-28. Constant lever device.

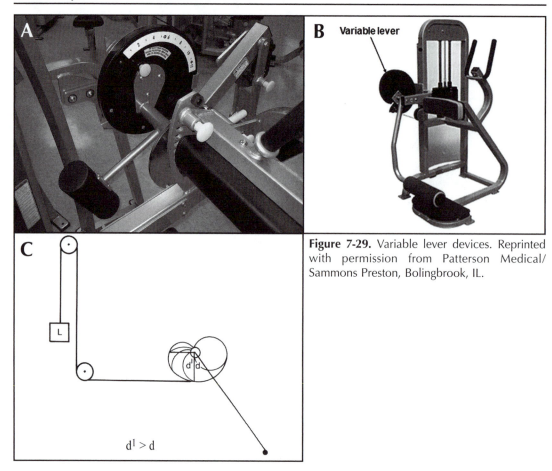

Figure 7-29. Variable lever devices. Reprinted with permission from Patterson Medical/Sammons Preston, Bolingbrook, IL.

The lever arm and the body part, however, change their position throughout the range of motion. This, in turn, changes the effect of gravity on them and affects the total resisting moment. The lever arm and body part may allow gravity to assist with the motion or may contribute to the resistance. The continuous lever may not be circular, but may be a cam with varying radii (Figure 7-29). The varying radii can be designed to allow for the effects of gravity on the body part and the lever system and the effects of changes in muscle length and angle of the muscle line of application. Such an arrangement can provide a maximum resisting moment throughout the entire range of motion. In the pulley system, the pulley arrangement may contain a moveable pulley (Figure 7-30). If so, remember the function of the moveable pulley (decreases the load by a factor of 2), and analyze its purpose within the exercise device.

CONTACT RESISTANCE

Strengthening exercises that use a force other than body weight all have a point of contact to transmit the magnitude of the load to the body part. However, this is not contact force as the actual resistance. A contact force as the resistance often occurs during isometric contractions when the body part is placed against an immoveable object and the individual contracts the muscle. The location of the contact provides the point of application, the line of application is perpendicular to the body part, and the direction opposes the attempted movement of the body part (Newton's Third Law). The magnitude is variable depending upon the force developed within the individual's muscle.

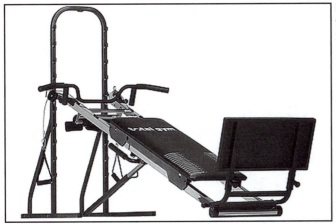

Figure 7-30. Pulley device. Reprinted with permission from Patterson Medical/ Sammons Preston, Bolingbrook, IL.

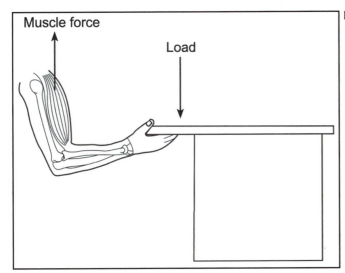

Muscle force

Load

Figure 7-31. Isometric contraction.

Example

For strengthening the elbow flexor muscles, a worker sitting upright at a desk may place both hands under the top of the desk with flexed elbows at the side of the chest. The worker then attempts to lift the desk (Figure 7-31). In this situation, the desk must be a greater load than the worker can move.

FRICTION

A few devices use friction as a resisting force ($F = \mu N$). A variety of configurations may occur. However, contact between a stationary surface and a rotating surface is common. The rotating surface is attached to a lever that provides a handle for the point of application (Figure 7-32). The line of application is perpendicular to the body part and the direction opposes the movement of the body part. The magnitude of the resisting force is adjusted by changing the normal force (N) on the device. The magnitude, however, may not be accurately provided in a quantitative value. The friction device allows for concentric contractions, and if the force of friction is large, it provides for isometric contractions. It does not allow for eccentric contractions. The shoulder wheel, the powder board, the weight sled, the upper body exerciser, and the stationary bicycle are examples of frictional devices (see Figure 7-32).

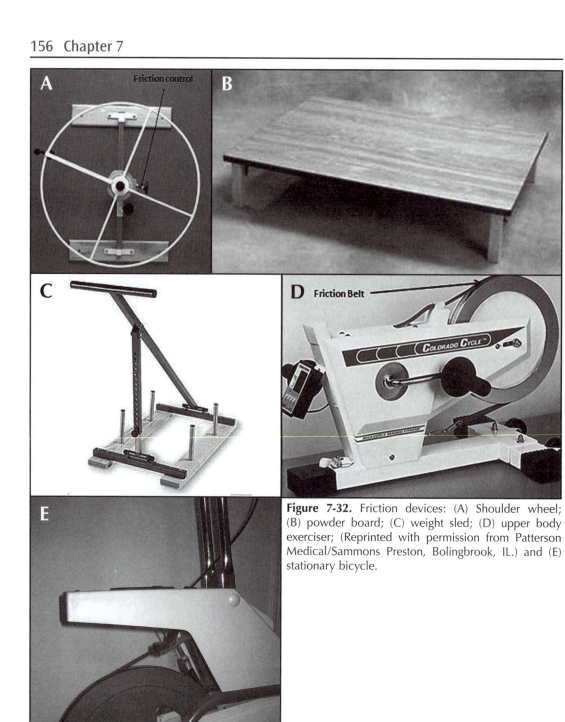

Figure 7-32. Friction devices: (A) Shoulder wheel; (B) powder board; (C) weight sled; (D) upper body exerciser; (Reprinted with permission from Patterson Medical/Sammons Preston, Bolingbrook, IL.) and (E) stationary bicycle.

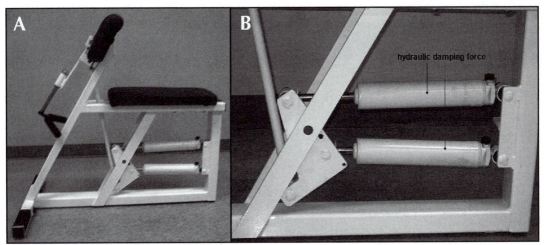

Figure 7-33. Hydraulic device.

Some frictional devices use the concept of "fluid friction" or viscosity to regulate resistance. The hydraulic cylinder is an example of this type of device (Figure 7-33). It is similar to the dashpot mentioned in Chapter 2. The device is a cylinder filled with fluid with an orifice or opening, through which fluid may escape. A lever system connected to the rod of the hydraulic device transmits the user's force to the cylinder. The resistance offered to the client depends upon the size of the orifice, the speed of motion, and the viscosity of the fluid. The user can adjust the resistance by turning a dial to change the size of the orifice or by changing the speed of motion. The resistance force (F) is related as

$$F \propto \eta v/A$$

where η is the coefficient of viscosity, v is the speed of movement, and A is the area of the orifice. The faster the client attempts to move, the greater the resistance is developed. Many brands of hydraulic exercise devices are available.

A gas has much less viscosity, which is increased as the gas is compressed. A pneumatic device that is based upon compressed gas allows the air in a cylinder to be compressed by a moving piston followed by an increase in the pressure within the cylinder. As the pressure is increased, the motion of the piston is opposed, tending to force the piston back in the opposite direction. The pneumatic device will provide resistance for concentric, eccentric, and isometric contractions. The Keiser line of equipment provides pneumatic resistance.

Muscular Resistance

For individuals (clients) with low strength, poor coordination, or limited joint stability, manual resistance may be necessary (Figure 7-34). A common procedure for manual resistance is proprioceptive neuromuscular facilitation (PNF). Muscle force from the person (clinician) providing the manual resistance is used as the load. The location of the hand contact is the point of application. The line of application is perpendicular to the body part; and the direction opposes the attempted movement of the individual's body part. The magnitude of the force is adjusted by the person applying the resistance. Usually, the magnitude of the resistance is not measured. However, a hand held dynamometer will provide an accurate value for the magnitude of force at the point of application (Figure 7-35). The type of contraction may be concentric, eccentric, or isometric depending upon the goals of the clinician. The clinician attempts to control the rate of the muscle contraction and the speed and direction of any movement.

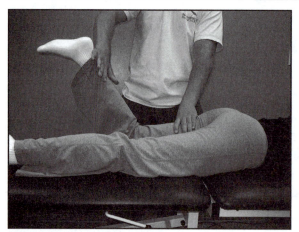

Figure 7-34. Manual resistance.

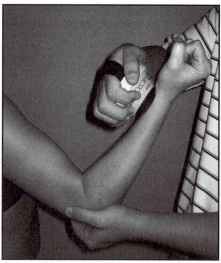

Figure 7-35. Resistance with a handheld dynamometer.

Example

For strengthening the muscle around the shoulder, the upper limb of the supine client is flexed and held at 90 degrees (Figure 7-36). This position reduces the effect of a gravitational moment. Manual resistance may be applied to the distal forearm perpendicular to the limb in any direction with a selected, but unmeasured, magnitude of force. The range of motion may be limited by the clinician's choice, and the clinician may stabilize the joint with the other hand. The variables in manual resistance are numerous. The point of application, line of application, direction, and magnitude of the resisting force may all be varied by the clinician. The body part may be positioned so that the force of gravity either assists or resists the client's muscle force. The clinician may choose to obtain any type of contraction response from the client.

INERTIAL RESISTANCE

Inertia is ubiquitous. A force is needed to start an object moving from a stationary position or to stop or change the direction of a moving object (Newton's First Law). The resisting force from inertia may come from any object with mass. The point of application may come through a pulley system, through a lever or combination of levers, or from direct contact with the object and the body part. The line of application may vary with the method of attachment to the body part, but the direction is opposite to the attempted movement of the body part. The magnitude of the resisting force depends upon the mass of the object and the acceleration ($F = ma$ and $T = I\alpha$). Concentric and eccentric contractions are related to inertial resistance. An isometric contraction occurs if the object does not move, but this situation was addressed in contact force as a resistance. The speed of movement (mv, $I\omega$) may vary from slow to as fast as the body part can move. The rate of force development may be minimal or explosive (Ft, Tt). Inertial resistance is usually used for training that involves a rapid change in contraction (Ft, Tt, and $P = \frac{W}{t}$) and motor learning. Examples of inertial exercise devices are the Impulse Inertial Device and leg weights (Figure 7-37).

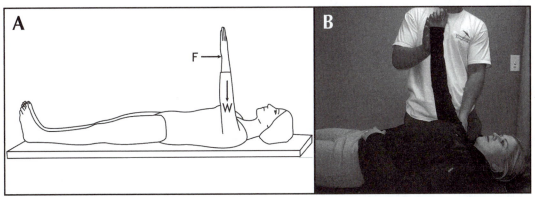

Figure 7-36. Manual resistance of the upper limb.

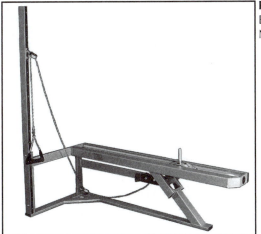

Figure 7-37. Inertial resistance on Impulse Inertial Exercise Trainer. (Courtesy of Impulse Training Systems, Newnan, GA.)

ELASTIC RESISTANCE

Elastic bands, cords, metal springs, and rods provide a resistance for strengthening exercises. As the strain of material increases, the resisting force increases ($F = -kl$). The point of application occurs where the material is attached to the body part or a hand piece. The line of application is along the line of the material or along a line of the attached pulley cord. As the body part moves through the range of motion, the pulley cord will change its angle with that body part. The magnitude depends upon the stiffness of the material and the amount of strain. The greater the stretch in the band or the bend in the rod, the greater the resistance will be. The load may be moved through a large range of motion concentrically and eccentrically or held in one position isometrically. The speed of movement may vary from slow to fast, and the rate of force development may be minimal or explosive.

Example

For strengthening the quadriceps muscles, an elastic band may be used (Figure 7-38). With the individual sitting on a chair, an elastic band is attached to the ankle at a 90-degree angle. Therefore, the line of application of the band is perpendicular to the leg, and its rotatory force component is maximum. Often, during this exercise, the leg travels from 90 degrees of knee flexion to full extension (0 degrees) and back to 90 degrees. As the limb travels through this range of motion, the line of application changes, which in turn reduces the percentage of the

Figure 7-38. Elastic resistance for the quadriceps muscles.

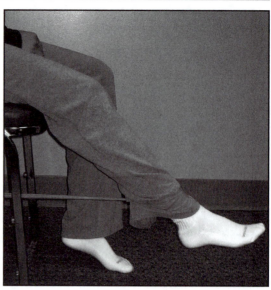

rotatory component by the sine of the angle the band makes with the leg. The combined segments of the leg and foot and the band provide the load to the quadriceps muscles. The quadriceps muscles shorten concentrically in the first part of the movement and lengthen during the return motion. The band increases in its length from 90 degrees of knee flexion to full extension, increasing its force. However, its rotatory component decreases. The gravitational force of the foot and leg provide an increase of resistance as the knee extends. Therefore, the magnitude of the load is the combined effects of the length of the band, the angle of the band with the limb, and the angle of the limb with the horizontal. The external load may be changed by using a band of a different stiffness (different color). The motion can emphasize concentric and eccentric without an isometric phase, or it may be predominantly isometric at any angle. The exercise may emphasize speed of movement by performing repetitions as quickly as possible, or it may be held isometrically for several seconds. The concentric contraction may be explosive or begin at a very slow rate.

BUOYANCY

Some exercises for individuals with very limited strength are performed in a pool (Figure 7-39). The buoyancy force of the water acts on the center of mass (point of application) of the body vertically (line of application) in an upward direction. The magnitude of the buoyant force (B) is equal to the weight of the water displaced by the body. The load on the feet during a squat in a pool would be the client's weight (W) minus the weight of the water displaced, or $F = W - B$ (see Figure 1-30). Note that the buoyant force on the body depends upon the amount of water that is displaced by the body. A client who begins a squat exercise in the pool with water waist high will have a decrease in load on the feet as the body is lowered into the squat position. The resisting moment for the quadriceps muscles would have a similar pattern as that of doing a squat with a barbell. However, the pattern would be modified by the buoyant effect of the water, which decreases the body weight component as the client performs the squat. The magnitude of the squat in a pool is definitely less than that of a squat with a barbell.

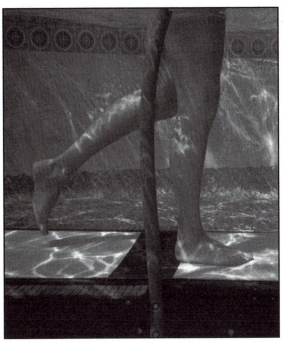

Figure 7-39. Buoyancy resistance. (© Ferno Aquatic Therapy, Wilmington, OH.)

ELECTROMAGNETIC RESISTANCE (EDDY CURRENTS)

Electromagnetic resistance is used in devices such as elliptical devices and stationary bicycles. Their effect on strength training is usually secondary to the effect upon cardiovascular and muscle endurance. The biomechanical factors involved in these devices take a lengthy discussion and will not be presented in this text.

Motion Analysis

Motion analysis and gait laboratories have been established to objectively analyze human motion. Objective measurement provided by motion analysis techniques is important to determine a client's progress or an athlete's improvement. Motion analysis involves measurements of anthropometrics, kinematics, and kinetics. Biomechanical analysis requires the use of anthropometric data such as body segment mass, segment lengths, segment centers of mass and moments of inertia, joint centers of rotation, and muscle point of application and line of application (see Appendix). The kinematic data include measured linear and rotatory displacements, duration of the movement, and calculated velocities and accelerations. Some accelerations may be directly measured by accelerometers. The kinetic data come directly from force plates and force transducers and are implied from muscle activation patterns (electromyography, or EMG).

Visual observation is very subjective, and some type of instrumentation that meets the criteria of a good measurement instrument (see Table 7-1) is needed to improve the accuracy of the data. Improvements in computer speed and memory capacity and improved software have made motion analysis more efficient for data collection, computation, analysis, and reporting. Advances in technology have allowed for synchronization of a variety of data collection devices. Methods for collecting objective data can range from using a stopwatch and foot markings to a sophisticated synchronized combination of video, force plate, and EMG analysis. All methods, however, use the biomechanical concepts included in this text.

Locomotion and Gait

Locomotion is the culmination of most of the concepts in the previous chapters. Entire books have been written on the description and analysis of locomotion and gait. Locomotion is defined as the translation of the body from one place to another and is evaluated in clinics and on the athletic field on a daily basis. Locomotion includes walking, running, stair ascent and descent, crawling, hopping, rolling a wheelchair, cycling, etc. Gait is generally defined as the manner of walking, but includes running and stair ascent and descent.

The translation of the body from one place to another during gait occurs because of rotatory motion of the limbs. The forces involved in gait are gravitational, inertial, muscular, and contact. These forces affect the displacement, velocity, and acceleration of the body and its individual segments.

The force of gravity acts on the body as a whole and on each individual segment. The point of application of this force is the center of mass (often referred to as the center of gravity) of the body and the center of mass of each segment. The line of application is vertical with a downward direction for the entire body and for each segment. The magnitude of the force is the weight of the total body or the weight of each segment.

Inertial force resists the change in motion of the body as a whole and also the movement of each individual segment. The moment of inertia is involved as the body segments rotate forward and backward on their axes.

Muscular forces control the motion caused by the interaction of the gravitational and inertial forces. The muscles provide force to the body segments that create moments around the joints. The muscular force comes from all of the muscles that are needed to accelerate and decelerate each body segment efficiently.

All forms of gait have contact with a supporting surface such as the ground, floor, stairs, etc. This contact establishes a reaction force that is usually referred to as a ground reaction force (GRF). The point of application of the GRF vector is referred to as the center of pressure. The GRF can be resolved into normal (perpendicular) and tangential components. The magnitude of these components depends upon the angle of the line of application of the combined forces of gravity and inertia as the foot contacts the surface. The magnitude is the combined gravitational and inertial forces of all of the body segments while the foot is in contact with the ground. With a more tangential component, the force of friction becomes more important. This importance of friction becomes evident as an individual walks on ice or starts to sprint. Contact forces are also involved within each joint (joint forces), especially in the weight-bearing joints. These joint forces are in response to the ground reaction and muscular forces and in a lesser part to inertial and gravitational forces.

Temporal and linear displacement of the entire body can be determined by simple methods such as a stopwatch, chalk, and a measuring tape. The variables considered include step time, step length, step width, foot angle, stride time, stride length, cadence, and walking and running velocity. Examples of such data include walking 30 ft in 1 min or running 100 m in 10 sec.

Other measures of linear and angular displacements of the body and body segments during gait take more sophisticated devices such as electrogoniometry or video. Some of the displacement variables determined are the linear motion of the center of mass of the body and excursion of joint angles. These movements determined in a certain time frame can provide values that allow calculations of velocities and accelerations. From these data, the inverse dynamics approach can be used to determine the net muscle moments. The equations of linear and angular motion can be applied to each body segment.

During gait, work is done to lift the center of mass of the body. As the center of mass rises, potential energy increases, and kinetic energy decreases. A very simple and rough method to estimate the path of the center of mass is to observe the movement of a point slightly anterior to the sacrum (level S2), and midway between the hips. The path of the instantaneous location of the center of mass of the body, however, is somewhat different than following such a point. As the body moves, the limbs change position, and this change affects the true location of the center of mass of the body. For example, a flexed limb raises the body's center of mass. Energy exchange occurs between each body segment. Therefore, an accurate determination of energy must include segmental energy exchange.

Activities

1. Define stability and balance.

2. List the characteristics that affect the stability of an object and explain how the principle of moments is involved with each.

3. Explain how individuals adjust their posture to improve stability in activities such as football or wrestling or during late-term pregnancy.

4. Describe and explain the differences among conventional, amputee, and basketball wheelchairs.

5. Analyze whether an individual while standing with his or her heels and back against a wall can stoop over to retrieve a $10 bill in front of his or her feet and return to the standing position without moving his or her feet.

6. Explain why the center of mass of an object should be near your center of mass when lifting or carrying the object.

7. Explain how the principle of moments can be used to determine the location of an individual's center of mass.

8. Explain how the principle of moments can be used to determine the weight of an individual's limb.

9. Describe the changes in the characteristics that affect stability as an individual performs a swing-through crutch gait.

10. Take a side view picture of an individual in a selected posture (eg, sitting and reaching toward the toes). From the picture, determine the location of the center of mass in that plane.

11. Does the center of mass of the body always lie within the body no matter what the position of the individual?

12. List the characteristics of a good test, and give an example of each.

13. Discuss the use of manual muscle testing as a method (instrument) to evaluate muscle strength based upon the criteria of a good measuring instrument.

14. Compare the exercise effect of various exercise devices.

15. List and evaluate devices that use the forces of gravity, contact, friction, muscular, inertia, elastic, buoyancy, and electromagnetic.

16. Analyze the mechanical factors involved in normal and abnormal gait.

Suggested Reading

Alcid JG, Ahmad CS, Lee TQ. Elbow anatomy and structural biomechanics. *Clin Sports Med.* 2004;23:503-517, vii.

Alkner BA, Tesch PA, Berg HE. Quadriceps EMG/force relationship in knee extension and leg press. *Med Sci Sports Exerc.* 2000;32:459-463.

Arampatzis A, De Monte G, Morey-Klapsing G. Effect of contraction form and contraction velocity on the differences between resultant and measured ankle joint moments. *J Biomech.* 2007;40:1622-1628.

Arjmand N, Shirazi-Adl A. Model and in vivo studies on human trunk load partitioning and stability in isometric forward flexions. *J Biomech.* 2006;39:510-521.

Arjmand N, Shirazi-Adl A. Role of intra-abdominal pressure in the unloading and stabilization of the human spine during static lifting tasks. *Eur Spine J.* 2006;15:1265-1275.

Banta JV. The evolution of gait analysis: a treatment decision-making tool. *Conn Med.* 2001;65:323-331.

Baudouin A, Hawkins D. A biomechanical review of factors affecting rowing performance. *Br J Sports Med.* 2002;36:396-402; discussion 402.

Bryce CD, Armstrong AD. Anatomy and biomechanics of the elbow. *Orthop Clin North Am.* 2008;39:141-154, v.

Budgeon MK, Latash ML, Zatsiorsky VM. Digit force adjustments during finger addition/removal in multi-digit prehension. *Exp Brain Res.* 2008;189:345-359.

Chambers HG, Sutherland DH. A practical guide to gait analysis. *J Am Acad Orthop Surg.* 2002;10:222-231.

Croce RV, Miller JP. Angle- and velocity-specific alterations in torque and semg activity of the quadriceps and hamstrings during isokinetic extension-flexion movements. *Electromyogr Clin Neurophysiol.* 2006;46:83-100.

Damavandi M, Barbier F, Leboucher J, Farahpour N, Allard P. Effect of the calculation methods on body moment of inertia estimations in individuals of different morphology. *Med Eng Phys.* 2009;31:880-886.

DesJardins JD, Walker PS, Haider H, Perry J. The use of a force-controlled dynamic knee simulator to quantify the mechanical performance of total knee replacement designs during functional activity. *J Biomech.* 2000;33:1231-1242.

Doheny EP, Lowery MM, Fitzpatrick DP, O'Malley MJ. Effect of elbow joint angle on force-EMG relationships in human elbow flexor and extensor muscles. *J Electromyogr Kinesiol.* 2008;18:760-770.

Doheny EP, Lowery MM, O'Malley MJ, Fitzpatrick DP. The effect of elbow joint centre displacement on force generation and neural excitation. *Med Biol Eng Comput.* 2009;47:589-598.

Durkin JL, Dowling JJ. Analysis of body segment parameter differences between four human populations and the estimation errors of four popular mathematical models. *J Biomech Eng.* 2003;125:515-522.

Durkin JL, Dowling JJ. Body segment parameter estimation of the human lower leg using an elliptical model with validation from DEXA. *Ann Biomed Eng.* 2006;34:1483-1493.

Erdemir A, Sirimamilla PA, Halloran JP, van den Bogert AJ. An elaborate data set characterizing the mechanical response of the foot. *J Biomech Eng.* 2009;131:094502.

Escamilla RF, Fleisig GS, Zheng N, et al. Effects of technique variations on knee biomechanics during the squat and leg press. *Med Sci Sports Exerc.* 2001;33:1552-1566.

Ferris DP, Gordon KE, Sawicki GS, Peethambaran A. An improved powered ankle-foot orthosis using proportional myoelectric control. *Gait Posture.* 2006;23:425-428.

Fleisig GS, Barrentine SW, Escamilla RF, Andrews JR. Biomechanics of overhand throwing with implications for injuries. *Sports Med.* 1996;21:421-437.

Gage WH, Winter DA, Frank JS, Adkin AL. Kinematic and kinetic validity of the inverted pendulum model in quiet standing. *Gait Posture.* 2004;19:124-132.

Gordon AM, Huxley AF, Julian FJ. The variation in isometric tension with sarcomere length in vertebrate muscle fibres. *J Physiol*. 1966;184:170-192.

Gordon KE, Sawicki GS, Ferris DP. Mechanical performance of artificial pneumatic muscles to power an ankle-foot orthosis. *J Biomech*. 2006;39:1832-1841.

Granata KR, Bennett BC. Low-back biomechanics and static stability during isometric pushing. *Hum Factors*. 2005;47:536-549.

Hansen EA, Lee HD, Barrett K, Herzog W. The shape of the force-elbow angle relationship for maximal voluntary contractions and sub-maximal electrically induced contractions in human elbow flexors. *J Biomech*. 2003;36:1713-1718.

Hodgins D. The importance of measuring human gait. *Med Device Technol*. 2008;19:42, 44-47.

Hooper DM, Hill H, Drechsler WI, Morrissey MC. Range of motion specificity resulting from closed and open kinetic chain resistance training after anterior cruciate ligament reconstruction. *J Strength Cond Res*. 2002;16:409-415.

Hooper DM, Morrissey MC, Drechsler W, Morrissey D, King J. Open and closed kinetic chain exercises in the early period after anterior cruciate ligament reconstruction. Improvements in level walking, stair ascent, and stair descent. *Am J Sports Med*. 2001;29:167-174.

Hsue BJ, Su FC. Gait and kinematics of the trunk and lower extremities in stair ascent using quadricane in healthy subjects. *Gait Posture*. 2009;29:146-150.

Jonkers I, Sauwen N, Lenaerts G, Mulier M, Van der Perre G, Jaecques S. Relation between subject-specific hip joint loading, stress distribution in the proximal femur and bone mineral density changes after total hip replacement. *J Biomech*. 2008;41:3405-3413.

Kawakami Y, Fukunaga T. New insights into in vivo human skeletal muscle function. *Exerc Sport Sci Rev*. 2006;34:16-21.

Kitaoka HB, Crevoisier XM, Hansen D, Katajarvi B, Harbst K, Kaufman KR. Foot and ankle kinematics and ground reaction forces during ambulation. *Foot Ankle Int*. 2006;27:808-813.

Koolstra JH, van Eijden TM. Biomechanical analysis of jaw-closing movements. *J Dent Res*. 1995;74:1564-1570.

Kuechle DK, Newman SR, Itoi E, Niebur GL, Morrey BF, An KN. The relevance of the moment arm of shoulder muscles with respect to axial rotation of the glenohumeral joint in four positions. *Clin Biomech (Bristol, Avon)*. 2000;15:322-329.

Lamontagne M, Beaulieu ML, Varin D, Beaule PE. Gait and motion analysis of the lower extremity after total hip arthroplasty: what the orthopedic surgeon should know. *Orthop Clin North Am*. 2009;40:397-405.

Latash ML, Gelfand IM, Li ZM, Zatsiorsky VM. Changes in the force-sharing pattern induced by modifications of visual feedback during force production by a set of fingers. *Exp Brain Res*. 1998;123:255-262.

Lunnen JD, Yack J, LeVeau BF. Relationship between muscle length, muscle activity, and torque of the hamstring muscles. *Phys Ther*. 1981;61:190-195.

Madigan ML, Davidson BS, Nussbaum MA. Postural sway and joint kinematics during quiet standing are affected by lumbar extensor fatigue. *Hum Mov Sci*. 2006;25:788-799.

Martinez-Villalpando EC, Herr H. Agonist-antagonist active knee prosthesis: a preliminary study in level-ground walking. *J Rehabil Res Dev*. 2009;46:361-373.

Mavroidis C, Nikitczuk J, Weinberg B, et al. Smart portable rehabilitation devices. *J Neuroeng Rehabil*. 2005;2:18.

Mesfar W, Shirazi-Adl A. Biomechanics of the knee joint in flexion under various quadriceps forces. *Knee*. 2005;12:424-434.

Nozaki D. Torque interaction among adjacent joints due to the action of biarticular muscles. *Med Sci Sports Exerc*. 2009;41:205-209.

Nozaki D, Nakazawa K, Akai M. Muscle activity determined by cosine tuning with a nontrivial preferred direction during isometric force exertion by lower limb. *J Neurophysiol*. 2005;93:2614-2624.

Ochs RM, Smith JL, Edgerton VR. Fatigue characteristics of human gastrocnemius and soleus muscles. *Electromyogr Clin Neurophysiol.* 1977;17:297-306.

Otis JC, Jiang CC, Wickiewicz TL, Peterson MG, Warren RF, Santner TJ. Changes in the moment arms of the rotator cuff and deltoid muscles with abduction and rotation. *J Bone Joint Surg Am.* 1994;76:667-676.

Ounpuu S. The biomechanics of walking and running. *Clin Sports Med.* 1994;13:843-863.

Peck CC, Hannam AG. Human jaw and muscle modelling. *Arch Oral Biol.* 2007;52:300-304.

Perry J, Burnfield JM. *Gait Analysis: Normal and Pathological Function.* 2nd ed. Thorofare, NJ: SLACK Incorporated; 2010.

Rassier DE, Herzog W. Force enhancement following an active stretch in skeletal muscle. *J Electromyogr Kinesiol.* 2002;12:471-477.

Rassier DE, MacIntosh BR, Herzog W. Length dependence of active force production in skeletal muscle. *J Appl Physiol.* 1999;86:1445-1457.

Riemer R, Hsiao-Wecksler ET. Improving net joint torque calculations through a two-step optimization method for estimating body segment parameters. *J Biomech Eng.* 2009;131:011007.

Schweizer A, Moor BK, Nagy L, Snedecker JG. Static and dynamic human flexor tendon-pulley interaction. *J Biomech.* 2009;42:1856-1861.

Senter C, Hame SL. Biomechanical analysis of tibial torque and knee flexion angle: implications for understanding knee injury. *Sports Med.* 2006;36:635-641.

Shelburne KB, Pandy MG, Torry MR. Comparison of shear forces and ligament loading in the healthy and ACL-deficient knee during gait. *J Biomech.* 2004;37:313-319.

Shelburne KB, Torry MR, Pandy MG. Contributions of muscles, ligaments, and the ground-reaction force to tibiofemoral joint loading during normal gait. *J Orthop Res.* 2006;24:1983-1990.

Shelburne KB, Torry MR, Pandy MG. Muscle, ligament, and joint-contact forces at the knee during walking. *Med Sci Sports Exerc.* 2005;37:1948-1956.

Shields RK, Madhavan S, Gregg E, et al. Neuromuscular control of the knee during a resisted single-limb squat exercise. *Am J Sports Med.* 2005;33:1520-1526.

Shimokochi Y, Shultz SJ. Mechanisms of noncontact anterior cruciate ligament injury. *J Athl Train.* 2008;43:396-408.

Smidt GL, Rogers MW. Factors contributing to the regulation and clinical assessment of muscular strength. *Phys Ther.* 1982;62:1283-1290.

Smith PA, Hassani S, Reiners K, Vogel LC, Harris GF. Gait analysis in children and adolescents with spinal cord injuries. *J Spinal Cord Med.* 2004;27 Suppl 1:S44-S49.

Tesch P, Karlsson J. Isometric strength performance and muscle fibre type distribution in man. *Acta Physiol Scand.* 1978;103:47-51.

Tsaopoulos DE, Baltzopoulos V, Richards PJ, Maganaris CN. In vivo changes in the human patellar tendon moment arm length with different modes and intensities of muscle contraction. *J Biomech.* 2007;40:3325-3332.

Wendlova J. Biomechanical conditions for maintaining body balance in kinesitherapy of osteoporotic patients. *Bratisl Lek Listy.* 2008;109:441-444.

Willardson JM. Core stability training: applications to sports conditioning programs. *J Strength Cond Res.* 2007;21:979-985.

Willardson JM, Fontana FE, Bressel E. Effect of surface stability on core muscle activity for dynamic resistance exercises. *Int J Sports Physiol Perform.* 2009;4:97-109.

Yu B, Garrett WE. Mechanisms of non-contact ACL injuries. *Br J Sports Med.* 2007;41 Suppl 1:i47-i51.

Appendix

System of Units

Various disciplines do not use the same systems of units. Although the International System of Units (SI) has become widely accepted, its use by practitioners in the United States is still not widespread. The loads in clinics and gyms are labeled in pounds, and the lengths and distances are in feet and inches. This is a basic text for practitioners and beginning researchers. Therefore, this edition will use the British Gravitational System. Because students may go beyond this text, and researchers and publications use SI units, conversions are presented in Table A-1.

Body Segment Characteristics

The estimation of body segment characteristics such as weight, center of mass, and mass moment of inertia is essential for calculating forces and moments on the body in the biomechanical analysis of postures and movements. The method of obtaining these values depends upon the time and finances available and the accuracy needed. The results obtained by Dempster,[1] Drillis and Contini,[2] Clauser and associates,[3] and Chandler and associates[4] are commonly presented in texts for the student or practitioner to quickly determine these forces and moments. These values, however, provide only estimates of the actual values and are not specific to an individual. They do not take into account the applicability of these values to several different populations. Tables A-2 and A-3 provide the estimations for weights and lengths needed to calculate forces, moments, and mass moments of inertia from various authors. The radius of gyration is needed to calculate the mass moment of inertia around the center of mass. In the body, however, a segment usually does not rotate around its center of mass. Therefore, the parallel axis theorem must be used to determine the radius of gyration from the proximal or distal end of the segment. From Dempster's moment of inertia data, Plagenhoef calculated the segmental radius of gyration about an axis perpendicular to the long axis of the body segment for the proximal and distal ends of each segment.[5] The mass moment of inertia (I) around the end of the segment (joint) is calculated by the equation $I = I_0 + mr^2$, where I_0 is the mass moment of inertia around the center of mass, m is the mass of the segment, and r is the length from the center of mass to the joint. Since $m = \frac{F}{a}$, the mass of a segment would be slugs = $lb/ft/sec^2$. Therefore, to determine the mass from the segment weight, the equation would be mass = segment weight/32.174 ft/sec^2, where 32.174 ft/sec^2 is the gravitational acceleration constant. The radii of gyration values are shown in Table A-3.

Table A-4 gives the average percent weight and weight and mass for a 150-lb man based upon adjusted values by Dempster.[1] Table A-5 provides values for principle moments of inertia converted to the British Gravitational System.

Determining the body segment characteristics of a specific individual can be time consuming and very expensive. Some researchers have taken measurements from the individual and then used linear and nonlinear regression equations and mathematical models to determine the segment values. Others have improved upon the board and scale method by using precise force plates to determine these values. A few have used invasive methods such as computerized tomography, magnetic resonance imaging, gamma radiation scanning, or dual energy X-ray absorptiometry (DEXA). Researchers may select one of these techniques to be more precise in their calculations.

TABLE A-1

Conversion Between the International System of Units (SI) and the British Gravitational System (BGS)

Item	SI to BGS	BGS to SI
Length	1 centimeter (cm) = 0.3937 inches (in)	1 in = 2.54 cm
	1 meter (m) = 39.37 in	1 ft =30.48 cm
	1 m = 3.281 feet (ft)	1 ft = 0.3048 m
	1 kilometer (km) = 0.621 mile (mi)	1 mi = 1.609 km
Area	1 cm^2 = 0.155 in^2	1 in^2 = 6.452 cm^2
	1 m^2 = 10.763 ft^2	1 ft^2 = 0.0929 m^2
Velocity	1 m/sec = 3.281 ft/sec	1 ft/sec = 0.3048 m/sec
	1 m/sec = 2.237 mi/hr	1 mi/hr =0.447 m/sec
Acceleration	1 m/sec^2 = 3.281 ft/sec^2	1 ft/sec^2 = 0.3048 m/sec^2
Mass	1 kilogram (kg) = 0.0683 slug	1 slug = 14.59 kg
Force	1 Newton (N) = 0.2248 pound (lb)	1 lb = 4.448 N
Torque	1 N • m = 0.7373 ft • lb	1 ft-lb = 1.3558 N • m
		1 kg$_f$ = 9.8 N
Mass moment of inertia	1 Kg • m^2 = 0.7373 slug • ft^2	1 slug • ft^2 = 1.356 K • gm^2
Angle	1 radian (rad) = 57.296 degrees	1 degree = 0.0175 radians
Pressure	1 Pascal (Pa) = 1 N/m^2 = 0.000147 lb/in^2 (psi)	1 psi = 6894.8 N/m^2 = 6894.8 Pa
Power	1 watt (Joules/sec) = 0.737 ft • lb/sec	1 ft • lb/sec = 1.356 watt
Work	1 Joule (J) = 0.737 ft • lb	1 ft • lb = 1.356 J

TABLE A-2

Link Boundaries (at Joint Centers) and Percentage Distance of Centers of Gravity from Link Boundaries

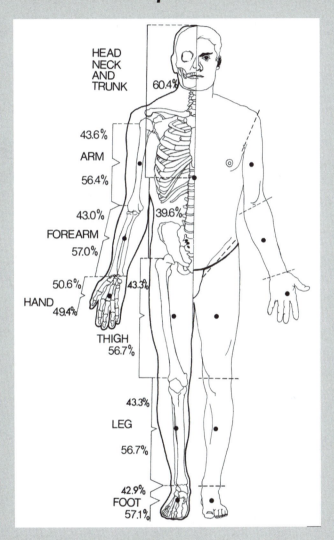

Data from Dempster WT. *Space Requirements of the Seated Operator: Geometrical, Kinematic, and Mechanical Aspects of the Body, With Special Reference to the Limbs.* Dayton, OH: WADC Technical Report 55-159; 1955.

TABLE A-3

Segmental Values for Percent Weight, Center of Mass, and Radius of Gyration

Source	Segmental Weight/Body Weight times 100			Center of Mass/Segment Length to Proximal End times 100			Radius of Gyration/Segment Length times 100	
	Dempster, 1955*	Drillis & Contini, 1966	Clauser et al, 1969	Dempster, 1955*	Drillis & Contini, 1966	Clauser et al, 1969	Plagenhoef, 1966, from Dempster's data	
							Proximal	Distal
Segment								
Head	8.1%	Head, neck, and trunk 58.04%	7.3%	43.3%		46.6%	Head, neck, and trunk 49.7%	Head, neck, and trunk 67.5%
Trunk	49.7		50.7	Thorax 62.7 Abd/pelvis 59.9		38.0		
Hand	0.6	0.6	0.7	50.6	39.2	48.0	58.7	57.7
Forearm	1.6	1.8	1.6	43.0	42.3	39.0	52.6	64.5
Forearm/hand	2.2	2.4	2.3	67.7	38.2	62.6	82.7†	56.5
Upper arm	2.8	3.57	2.6	43.6	44.9	51.3	54.2	64.5
Upper limb	5	5.97	4.9	51.2	43.1	41.3	64.5‡	59.6
Foot	1.4	1.35	1.5	24.9 to ankle axis 43.8 to heel	to heel 44.5	44.9	69.0	69.0
Leg	4.6	4.2	4.3	43.3	39.3	37.1	52.8	64.3
Leg/foot	6.1	5.55	5.8	43.4	45.0	47.5	73.5‡	57.2
Thigh	9.9	9.46	10.3	43.3	41.0	37.2	54.0	65.3
Lower limb	16.1	15.01	16.1	43.4	39.7	38.2	56.0‡	65.0
Total body						41.2		

*adjusted values
†to ulnar styloid
‡to medial malleolus

TABLE A-4

Average Percent Weight, and Weight and Mass for 150-lb Man*

Body Part	% Weight	Weight (lb)	Mass (slugs)	Weight (N)	Mass (kg)
Total	100	150	4.6583	667.5	68.003
Hand	0.6	0.9	0.0280	4.005	0.408
Forearm	1.6	2.4	0.0745	10.680	1.088
Forearm/hand	2.2	3.3	0.1025	14.685	1.496
Upper arm	2.8	4.2	0.1304	18.690	1.904
Upper limb	5	7.5	0.2329	33.375	3.400
Head	8.1	12.15	0.3773	54.068	5.508
Trunk	49.7	74.55	2.3152	331.748	33.796
Thigh	9.9	14.85	0.4612	66.083	6.732
Leg	4.6	6.9	0.2143	30.705	3.128
Foot	1.4	2.1	0.0652	9.345	0.952
Leg/foot	6.1	9.15	0.2842	40.718	4.148
Lower limb	16.1	24.15	0.7500	107.468	10.948

*mass = segment weight/32.174 ft/s

Based upon adjusted values from Dempster WT. *Space Requirements of the Seated Operator: Geometrical, Kinematic, and Mechanical Aspects of the Body, With Special Reference to the Limbs.* Dayton, OH: WADC Technical Report 55-159; 1955.

TABLE A-5

Principle Moments of Inertia (Slug • in²)

Segment	I_{cm} $X \pm s$	I_o $X \pm s$
Head and neck	3.12 ± 0.66	15.07 ± 2.85*
Thorax	12.26 ± 0.60	41.23 ± 17.95†
Abdominal-pelvic region	46.07 ± 33.27	77.18 ± 38.94‡
Arm	1.49 ± 0.48	4.33 ± 1.54
Forearm	0.59 ± 0.10	1.94 ± 0.50
Hand	0.05 ± 0.02	3.22 ± 0.08
Upper limb	11.04 ± 2.81	36.08 ± 10.98
Forearm/hand	2.02 ± 0.54	6.26 ±1.61
Thigh	11.58 ± 9.18	31.84 ± 12.71
Leg	4.50 ± 1.53	14.93 ± 6.39
Foot	0.32 ± 0.05	6.86 ± 0.28
Lower limb	73.34 ± 21.18	193.08 ± 62.69
Leg/foot	11.44 ± 4.01	35.40 ± 12.14

*From hip joint; †From TI2 vertebra; ‡From C7 vertebra

Data from Dempster WT. *Space Requirements of the Seated Operator: Geometrical, Kinematic, and Mechanical Aspects of the Body, With Special Reference to the Limbs.* Dayton, OH: WADC Technical Report 55-159; 1955.

References

1. Dempster WT. *Space Requirements of the Seated Operator: Geometrical, Kinematic, and Mechanical Aspects of the Body, With Special Reference to the Limbs.* Dayton, OH: WADC Technical Report 55-159; 1955.

2. Drillis R, Contini R. *Body segment parameters.* DHEW 1166-03. New York University, School of Engineering and Science; 1966.

3. Clauser CE, McConville JT, Young JW. *Weight, volume, and center of mass of segments of the human body.* AMRL-TR-69-70. Dayton, OH: Wright-Patterson Air Force Base; 1969.

4. Chandler RF, Clauser CE, McConville JT, Reynolds HM, Young JW. *Investigation of inertial properties of the human body.* DOT HS-801430. Dayton, OH: Wright-Patterson Air Force Base; 1975.

5. Plagenhoef SC. Methods of obtaining kinetic data to analyze human motions. *The Research Quarterly of the American Association for Health, Physical Education, and Recreation.* 1966;37(1):103-112.

Suggested Reading

Bauer JJ, Pavol MJ, Snow CM, Hayes WC. MRI-derived body segment parameters of children differ from age-based estimates derived using photogrammetry. *J Biomech.* 2007;40(13):2904-2910.

Bjornstrup J. Estimation of human body segment parameters—statistical analysis of results from prior investigations, Technical report, Lab of Image Analysis, Institute of Electronic Systems, Aalborg University; 1995.

Damavandi M, Farahpour N, Allard P. Determination of body segment masses and centers of mass using a force plate method in individuals of different morphology. *Medical Engineering & Physics.* 2009:31.

Davidson PL, Wilson SJ, Wilson BD, Chalmers DJ. Estimating subject-specific body segment parameters using a 3-dimensional modeller program. *J Biomech.* 2008;41(16):3506-3510.

Durkin JL, Dowling JJ. Analysis of body segment parameter differences between four human populations and the estimation errors of four popular mathematical models. *J Biomech Eng.* 2003;125(4):515-523.

Hanavan EP. *A mathematical model of the human body.* AMRL-TR-64-102. Dayton, OH: Wright-Patterson Air Force Base; 1964.

Huang HK, Suarez FR. Evaluation of cross sectional geometry and mass density distributions of humans and laboratory animals using computerized tomography. *J Biomech.* 1983;16:821-832.

Lee MK, Le NS, Fang AC, Koh MTH. Measurement of body segment parameters using dual energy X-ray absorptiometry and three-dimensional geometry: An application in gait analysis. *J Biomech.* 2009;42(3):217-222.

Lenzi D, Cappello A, Chiari L. Influence of body segment parameters and modeling assumptions on the estimate of center of mass trajectory. *J Biomech.* 2003;36(9):1335-1341.

Miller DI, Nelson RC. *Biomechanics of Sport.* Philadelphia, PA: Lea & Febiger; 1973.

Nikolova GS, Toshev YE. Estimation of male and female body segment parameters of the Bulgarian population using a 16-segmental mathematical model. *J Biomech V.* 2007;40(16):3700-3707.

Pavol MJ, Owings TM, Grabiner MD. Body segment inertial parameter estimation for the general population of older adults. *J Biomech.* 2002;35(5):707-712

Park SJ, Kim C-B, Park SC. Anthropometric and biomechanical characteristics on body segments of Koreans. *Appl Human Sci.* 1999;18(3):91-99.

Pataky TC, Zatsiorsky VM, Challis JH. A simple method to determine body segment masses in vivo: reliability, accuracy and sensitivity analysis. *Clinical Biomechanics.* 2003;18(4):364-368.

Pavol MJ, Owings TM, Grabiner MD. Body segment inertial parameter estimation for the general population of older adults. *J Biomech.* 2002;35(5):707-712.

Plagenhoef S, Evans FG, Abdelnour T. Anatomical data for analyzing human motion. *Res Q Exercise Sport.* 1983;54:169-178.

Schneider K, Zernicke RF. Mass, center of mass, and moment of inertia estimates for infant limb segments. *J Biomech.* 1992;25(2):145-148.

Shan G, Bohn C. Anthropometrical data and coefficients of regression related to gender and race. *Applied Ergonomics*. 2003;34:327-337.

Winter DA. *Biomechanics and Motor Control of Human Movement*. 4th ed. Hoboken, NJ: John Wiley & Sons; 2004.

Zatsiorsky VM. *Kinetics of Human Motion*. Champaign, IL: Human Kinetics; 2002.

Zatsiorsky VM, Seluyanov VN. The mass and inertia characteristics of the main segments of the human body. In Matsui H, Kobayashi K, Eds. *Biomechanics VIII-B*. Champaign, IL: Human Kinetics; 1983:1152-1159.

Zatsiorsky VM, Seluyanov VN. Estimation of the mass and inertia characteristics of the human body by means of the best predictive regression equations. In Winter DA, Norman RW, Wells RP, Hayes KC, and Patla AE, Eds. *Biomechanics IX-B*. Champaign, IL: Human Kinetics. 1985:233-239.

Index